Sterilization and Disinfection for the Perioperative Nurse

Guest Editor

TERRI GOODMAN, PhD, RN, CNOR

PERIOPERATIVE NURSING CLINICS

www.periopnursing.theclinics.com

Consulting Editor
NANCY GIRARD, PhD, RN, FAAN

September 2010 • Volume 5 • Number 3

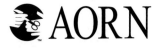

SAUNDERS an imprint of ELSEVIER, Inc.

W.B. SAUNDERS COMPANY

A Division of Elsevier Inc.

1600 John F. Kennedy Boulevard • Suite 1800 • Philadelphia, Pennsylvania 19103-2899

http://www.periopnursing.theclinics.com

PERIOPERATIVE NURSING CLINICS Volume 5, Number 3
September 2010 ISSN 1556-7931, ISBN-13: 978-1-4377-2481-3

Editor: Katie Hartner

Perioperative Nursing Clinics (ISSN 1556-7931) is published quarterly by Elsevier, 360 Park Avenue South, New York, NY 10010. Months of issue are March, June, September and December. Business and Editorial Offices: 1600 John F. Kennedy Blvd., Suite 1800, Philadelphia, PA 19103-2899. Customer Service Office: 11830 Westline Industrial Drive, St. Louis, MO 63146. Periodicals postage paid at New York, NY and at additional mailing offices. Subscription prices are $116.00 per year (domestic individuals), $213.00 per year (domestic institutions), $58.00 per year (domestic students/residents), $150 per year (international individuals), $245 per year (international institutions), and $62.00 per year (International students/residents). Foreign air speed delivery is included in all *Clinics* subscription prices. All prices are subject to change without notice. **POSTMASTER:** Send change of address to *Perioperative Nursing Clinics*, Customer Service (orders, claims, online, change of address): Elsevier Periodicals Customer Service, 11830 Westline Industrial Drive, St. Louis, MO 63146. Tel: 1-800-654-2452 (U.S. and Canada). Fax: 314-523-5170. E-mail: journalscustomerservice-usa@elsevier.com (for print support); journalsonlinesupport-usa@elsevier.com (for online support).

Reprints. For copies of 100 or more, of articles in this publication, please contact the Commercial Rights Department, Elsevier Inc., 360 Park Avenue South, New York, NY 10010-1710; Phone: (+1) 212-633-3813; Fax: (+1) 212-462-1935; E-mail: reprints@elsevier.com.

Printed in the United States of America.

Contributors

CONSULTING EDITOR

NANCY GIRARD, PhD, RN, FAAN
Consultant, Boerne; Clinical Associate Professor, Acute Nursing Care Department,
University of Texas Health Science Center, San Antonio, Texas

GUEST EDITOR

TERRI GOODMAN, PhD, RN, CNOR
Terri Goodman & Associates, Dallas, Texas

AUTHORS

CHERI ACKERT-BURR, RN, MSN, CNOR
Clinical Specialist, TSO3, Dalton, Quebec, Canada

PAMELA CARTER, RN, BSN, CNOR
Clinical Education Specialist, STERIS Corporation, Mentor, Ohio

NANCY CHOBIN, RN, AAS, ACSP, CSPDM
Sterile Processing Educator, Saint Barnabas Healthcare System, West Orange,
New Jersey

LINDA CLEMENT, BSM, CRCST
Consumable Territory Manager, STERIS Corporation, Mentor, Ohio

SUSAN CLOUSER, RN, MSN, CRNO
Plano, Texas

LYNDA D. DOELL, MSN, RN, CIC, CPHQ
Infection Prevention Coordinator, Infection Prevention, Plano, Texas

JUDITH LIPTON GOLDBERG, MSN, RN, CNOR, CRCST
Clinical Director, Sterile Processing Department, The William W. Backus Hospital,
Norwich, Waterford, Connecticut

NYLA "SKEE" JAPP, RN, PhD, CSPDM
Professional Central Sterile Processing Department Training and Mentoring,
Phoenix, Arizona

M. CHRIS KING, RN, CRCST
Clinical Education Specialist, STERIS Corporation, Mentor, Ohio

CARLA MCDERMOTT, RN, BS, CNOR, CRCST
Baycare Healthcare System, South Florida Baptist Hospital, Plant City, Florida

PATRICIA A. MEWS, RN, MHA, CNOR
Management Consultant, Mews Surgical Consulting, Scottsdale, Arizona

LIZ STONEMAN, RN, BSN
Vice President, Sales Team Development, Ascent Healthcare Solutions, Phoenix, Arizona

MICHELLE R. TINKHAM, RN, BSN, PHN, MS, CNOR, CLNC, RNFA
General/Vascular/Trauma Resource Nurse, Riverside Community Hospital, Riverside, California

MARTHA L. YOUNG, BS, MS, LLC
President Martha L. Young, SAVVY Sterilization Solutions, Woodbury, Minnesota

Contents

> In the perioperative arena, a solid understanding of cleaning, disinfection, and sterilization processes is essential for nurses to be effective in their role as patient advocates. Patient safety is enhanced when perioperative nurses have knowledge that extends beyond the basics of these procedures. This article provides a concise overview of the information on cleaning, disinfection, and sterilization contained in the Association of Perioperative Registered Nurses Recommended Practices that affects the work of the perioperative nurse on a daily basis.

> Sterilization of instruments and devices is a complex process; improperly processed instruments and devices can be very detrimental to patient safety. Success includes the education and effective participation of everyone who handles instruments from one point of use to the next, which includes the perioperative staff as well as those who work in the central sterile processing department. This article describes high-temperature sterilization and the various sterilizers available. Special focus is on sterilizing instruments that have come in contact with patients with Creutzfeldt-Jakob disease.

> Nurses in surgical settings have responsibility for protecting patient and staff safety on a tight budget. This responsibility includes having current knowledge of the process, efficacy, safety, and cost of a variety of sterilization methods. Using low-temperature sterilization technologies and following regulatory mandates pose challenges for the perioperative nurse. This article provides information to guide the nurse in making informed decisions concerning low-temperature sterilization of surgical instrument processing.

> The process of flash sterilization has evolved since its inception. The process of flash sterilization continues to evolve focusing on what is needed to

guarantee that flash sterilization is safe, effective and will ultimately ensure patient safety and reduce surgical site infections. Today's practice is more complex with the necessity for increased knowledge and staff competencies of the entire sterilization process. The way that regulatory agencies review or assess a facility's process for flash sterilization is also changing. The sterilization processes are assessed to ensure that they deliver safe products for patients. Because of the increased incidences of surgical site infections and health care–associated infections, it is imperative that all steps of the sterilization process be followed consistently and conscientiously. Flash sterilization can be a safe and effective process for the sterilization of instruments intended for immediate use during operative/invasive procedures. Perioperative managers should review and audit current practices and implement a workable, continuous, quality-improvement program.

The goal of perioperative registered nurse is to minimize patient risk for surgical site infection. This goal can be achieved by keeping up-to-date on the recommended procedures that establish the clinical practice for improving the outcome of the steam sterilization process. This improvement involves development and adherence to policies and procedures, training, competency testing, and ongoing education to eliminate operator errors, which are the primary reason for a sterilization process failure. This article discusses why and how the steam sterilization process should be monitored so that medical devices not properly sterilized do not contact the patient.

Disinfection and sterilization practices are regulated and monitored by several agencies, both voluntary and mandatory. The practice of adequate disinfection and sterilization affects every surgical patient. Process failures can have debilitating lifelong effects. Education of administrators and managers through frontline workers helps ensure compliance with standards, regulations, and statutes whose goals are aligned with every perioperative nurse in providing safe, evidence-based, high-quality health care.

Infection prevention in the perioperative arena requires collaboration between the perioperative nurse and the infection preventionist. This article presents key concepts, processes, expected outcomes, possible barriers, and strategies to prevent surgical site infections and staff exposures in the perioperative health care setting from an infection prevention perspective.

Susan Clouser

Toxic anterior segment syndrome (TASS) is an acute, sterile inflammation of the anterior chamber of the eye after an intraocular procedure. There are many possible causes of TASS, but the majority of cases result from inadequate instrument cleaning, transfer of particulate matter, especially on the intraocular lens, and preservatives in medications. Paying strict attention to these key areas prevents TASS in most cases.

THE CLINICS ARE NOW AVAILABLE ONLINE!

Access your subscription at:
www.theclinics.com

Preface

Like surgery, the processing of surgical instruments and devices is a team sport. Although it is usually the sterile processing department (SPD) that prepares instruments and devices for surgical procedures, the perioperative nurse has a definite impact on both process and outcomes. A thorough understanding of the principles and practice of sterilization and disinfection is integral to delivering safe patient care in the operating room.

It is the sterile environment that makes the operating room a unique patient care area, and knowledge is key to making appropriate decisions about the surgical instruments and devices used in procedures. Patient safety depends on the perioperative nurse's ability to protect the sterile field and to assure that anything that should be sterile *is*, in fact, sterile. It is also important to facilitate clinical sustainability by preventing costly damage by ensuring that instruments and devices are managed properly.

Participating in the sterilization/disinfection process can be as simple as ensuring that instruments are not returned to the SPD covered with dried blood and bioburden. Items must be clean before they can be sterilized, and the more difficult it is to clean an item, the greater the potential that it will not be sterile. "You can clean without sterilizing, but you can't sterilize without cleaning"—a simple but important concept.

Good communication with the SPD includes the proper sorting of instruments being returned for processing and clearly identifying any instrument or device that is not functioning properly so that it will not be returned to the operating room unrepaired. More complex participation requires understanding how delicate and intricate items must be processed and recognizing the variety of sterility monitoring devices, to be sure that each item was processed appropriately.

Even in biblical times, it seems, they understood the concept of clean and sterile. God instructed Moses: "Anything else that can withstand fire must be put through the fire, and then it will be clean. But it must also be purified with the water of cleansing. And whatever cannot withstand fire must be put through that water." Numbers 31:23.

This issue of *Perioperative Nursing Clinics* is to serve as a resource for the perioperative nurse to improve practice and ensure patient safety in the sterile environment by first understanding the essential role that the perioperative nurse plays in the processing and sterilization of instruments and supplies.

Terri Goodman, PhD, RN, CNOR
Terri Goodman & Associates
PO Box 29133
Dallas, TX 75229, USA

E-mail address:
terrigoodman@sbcglobal.net

Perioperative Nursing Clinics 5 (2010) xi
doi:10.1016/j.cpen.2010.06.001

What the Perioperative Nurse Needs to Know About Cleaning, Disinfection, and Sterilization

Judith Lipton Goldberg, MSN, RN, CNOR, CRCST[a,b]

KEYWORDS

• Sterilization • Disinfection • Education • Perioperative

Perioperative nurses are patient advocates. These nurses are responsible for patient safety through careful and appropriate assessment, planning, interventions, and the evaluation of outcomes. In the perioperative arena, a solid understanding of cleaning, disinfection, and sterilization processes is essential for nurses to be effective in their role as patient advocates. Patient safety is enhanced when perioperative nurses have knowledge that extends beyond the basics of cleaning, disinfection and sterilization.

In addition to being intimately familiar with the methods of sterilization available in their workplaces, patient advocates must be aware of the wide variety of additional sterilization methods available today. Advocates must understand how the variety of mechanical, chemical, and biologic indicators and integrators that are used in the facility work, and must be able to interpret the results of monitoring. Nurses must be able to differentiate between flash and terminal sterilization and understand the implications of each approach. Safe patient care includes the ability to properly select and use the various choices for instrument containment, for example, rigid containers, outside wraps, and peel pouches. For instance, the effective perioperative nurse knows why peel pouches are not safe to use within a wrapped instrument set or rigid container. Perioperative nurses need to know the importance of following manufacturers' instructions and understand that those instructions may change and must be updated with each new product they receive.

Current knowledge, experience, and evidence-based practices are the cornerstones of good decision-making. Many appropriate decisions made in the operating room are indisputable; others are not as obvious, creating the potential for making

[a] Sterile Processing Department, The William W. Backus Hospital, Norwich, CT, USA
[b] 91 Braman Road, Waterford, CT 06385, USA
E-mail address: goldbem@msn.com

Perioperative Nursing Clinics 5 (2010) 263–272
doi:10.1016/j.cpen.2010.04.009
1556-7931/10/$ – see front matter © 2010 Elsevier Inc. All rights reserved.

poor choices that may put patients at risk for infection. Perioperative nurses should have a working knowledge of the specific Association of Perioperative Registered Nurses (AORN) Recommended Practices related to cleaning, disinfection, and sterilization.

This article provides a concise overview of the information contained in recommended practices that affects the work of the perioperative nurse on a daily basis. The 6 AORN Recommended Practices that focus on cleaning, disinfection, and sterilization include:

- Cleaning, handling, and processing anesthesia equipment
- High-level disinfection
- Cleaning and processing flexible endoscopes and endoscope accessories
- Cleaning and care of surgical instruments and powered equipment
- Selection and use of packaging systems for sterilization
- Sterilization in the perioperative practice setting.[1–6]

CLEANING, HANDLING, AND PROCESSING ANESTHESIA EQUIPMENT

Perioperative nurses are often involved with anesthesia equipment. The nurses assist anesthesia providers during patient induction and emergence and during procedures. Nurses managing patients with moderate sedation are responsible for the anesthesia equipment they are using. Therefore, nurses should be aware that "anesthesia equipment that comes in contact with mucous membranes should be sterilized or undergo high-level disinfection before use."[1(p569)] Nurses should work with members of the anesthesia department to ensure that items used for patient care are processed according to the manufacturer's recommendations.

Following is a situation that caused confusion, anger, and disappointment, and could have resulted in harm to a patient because product information was not reviewed prior to purchase. New laryngoscope blades were purchased and sent to sterile processing for high-level disinfection, assuming they would be processed in the same manner as older models familiar to the staff. However, a review of the manufacturer's instructions for the product clearly indicated that the new blades could not be high-level disinfected and required terminal sterilization. Such a situation would be avoided if all new products and product literature were reviewed prior to purchase.

HIGH-LEVEL DISINFECTION

Although most items used in the operating room will be terminally sterilized, there are some that require high-level disinfection. Items to be processed are classified into 3 categories—critical, semicritical, and noncritical—based on the Spaulding classification system.[2(p579–586)] Items in all categories must be cleaned before sterilization or disinfection. Critical items enter sterile tissue and must be terminally sterilized; semicritical items are exposed to mucous membranes or nonintact skin and require high-level disinfection; and noncritical items contact only intact skin and require only low-level disinfection. Disinfected and sterilized items must be appropriately protected during transport.

Ultrasound probes and bougie dilators must be high-level disinfected. Ultrasound probes are typically draped before use but some, such as laparoscopic and neurosurgical probes, enter sterile body cavities. Should these particular probes be terminally sterilized or high-level disinfected? These decisions should be made by facilities after carefully reviewing the products, their intended use, and the manufacturer's instructions for cleaning, disinfection, and sterilization. In some instances, even if a facility would prefer to terminally sterilize these probes, there may not be containers or packaging systems large enough to accommodate their length or shape. When a facility has a sterilization committee, these complex issues should be referred to the committee for review and recommendations. At the very least, the facility infection preventionist should be consulted for input.

CLEANING AND PROCESSING FLEXIBLE ENDOSCOPES AND ENDOSCOPE ACCESSORIES

Flexible endoscopes and endoscope accessories should be precleaned at the point of use.[3(p596)] Precleaning with an enzymatic detergent before transport to the decontamination and reprocessing area prevents debris from drying both inside the channels and on the outside of the endoscope. Based on several research studies, the AORN now recommends that all flexible endoscopes be reprocessed if more than 5 days have passed since the last processing.[3(p601)] Facilities should develop systems to identify scopes that need to be reprocessed, and educate staff to implement the system as well as to check scope outdates before selecting one for use. Policies addressing the processing and labeling of scopes should be reviewed by sterile processing and infection control, and should be applied consistently in all departments in the facility that handle flexible endoscopes. Staff handling flexible endoscopes should be trained in the care and handling of the scopes and should demonstrate competency on a scheduled basis. Initial training should occur, followed by updates when manufacturer instructions change or recommended practices are updated and revised.

CLEANING AND CARE OF SURGICAL INSTRUMENTS AND POWERED EQUIPMENT

Newly purchased instruments, items returned from repair, and loaner or consignment instrumentation should be cleaned and inspected before sterilization.[4(p611–612)] In many facilities, instruments are delivered directly to the operating room to save time; this is a dangerous shortcut and can put patients at risk for surgical site infections. Perioperative nurses should be aware that it is imperative that all instrumentation and devices, even those thought to be decontaminated or sterilized by other organizations or at a manufacturer facility, be disassembled and thoroughly inspected before terminal processing in the facility.

Complex items can be very difficult to clean and to sterilize, so it is essential to have complete manufacturer's instructions available. Instructions initially should be reviewed by at least 2 sterile processing personnel and the vendor representative to ensure understanding and compliance. Patient safety is at risk every time instructions are not received or not followed. Perioperative nurses and surgical technologists should also have this information prior to using new items. Working together with vendors, operating room personnel, and sterile processing staff can greatly decrease errors in processing and reduce delays in surgery.[7] If manufacturer's instructions are not obtained or not followed, the organization assumes risk and the manufacturer is released from any liability.[8]

Instruments and devices that contain bioburden cannot be disinfected or sterilized. Allowing blood or body fluids to dry on the surface and inside of instruments can lead to the transmission of infections. "Instruments should be kept free of gross soil during surgical procedures."[4(p613)] During a surgical procedure, instruments should be wiped with a sterile water-soaked sponge or submerged in a basin of water.[9] Use of saline to soak or wipe instruments can lead to pitting, rusting, and corrosion, and can shorten instrument life. Instruments with lumens should be flushed during and following the procedure to prevent obstruction. "To prevent aerosolization, the scrub person should keep the instrument below the surface of the water when irrigating it."[9(p538)] In addition to wiping instruments of gross contamination during a procedure, it is critical that items be soaked or sprayed with an enzymatic cleaner that can begin to break down blood and body fluids prior to entering the sterile processing department. "Instruments should be treated with an instrument cleaner....before transport.[4(p614)]" Instruments can also be wrapped or covered with towels soaked with water to keep them moist.

Cleaning always begins at the point of use of the instrumentation; gross soil and debris must be removed at the point of use. "Cleaning and decontamination should occur as soon as possible after instruments and equipment are used."[4(p613),10] Hinged instruments should be opened; heavy instruments should be separated from light ones; and sharp instruments that might cause injury to a sterile processing employee should be set apart. "Lightweight instruments should be placed on top of heavier instruments or segregated into separate containers."[4(p614)]

Delays in the reprocessing of instruments and priority items can lead to costly delays in surgery. It is critical that priority instruments are identified to alert sterile processing personnel that they are needed more quickly than the usual turnaround time. However, the minimum turnaround time of items is determined by the time it takes to properly process them: cleaning, disinfecting, hand washing delicate items, using the sonic washer for complex instrumentation, drying instrument containers if required by the method of sterilization, inspecting instruments for cleanliness and functionality, and the cooling time required after steam sterilization.

SELECTION AND USE OF PACKAGING SYSTEMS FOR STERILIZATION

Packaging systems should be selected as appropriate to the method of sterilization the items require.[5(p637–638)] Package selection should also include ergonomic considerations. The total weight of a containerized set should not exceed 25 pounds (11.34 kg), considering the safety of staff in both sterile processing and in the operating room. Agencies such as Association for the Advancement of Medical Instrumentation (AAMI) and Association of Perioperative Registered Nurses (AORN) have recommended this. There is also the possibility that sterility may be compromised due to the complexity and weight of sets greater than 25 pounds. Peel pouches may not be used within a wrapped or containerized set because the position of the pouch during sterilization can prevent air removal and penetration of the sterilant and concerns about adequate drying.[5(p640)] Peel pouch manufacturers have not validated their pouches for use in instrument sets.[9] There are rigid containers of various shapes and sizes designed to hold small items as well as commercially available paper bags that have been validated for use within sets. Disposable paper filters in rigid containers should always be checked for integrity before the instruments are used in the operating room.

STERILIZATION IN THE PERIOPERATIVE PRACTICE SETTING

There are many regulatory requirements for sterilization, including federal, state, and professional associations that guide practice. Agencies such as Centers for Medicare and Medicaid Services (CMS), The Joint Commission, Departments of Public Health (DPH), AAMI, AORN, and the American National Standards Organization (ANSI) all have recommendations and requirements that influence practice. It is important that operating room staff is aware of these guiding principles and requirements, especially if there are sterilizers in the operating rooms that are operated by the nursing and technologist staff or by support staff.[11] With the increase in ambulatory surgical centers perioperative nurses are increasingly responsible for the processing of instruments, including sterilization. This processing requires the same procedures and regulations as a sterile processing department.[9]

Gravity displacement and dynamic air-removal sterilization are 2 methods of steam sterilization used for items that can tolerate moisture and heat. In a gravity displacement sterilizer, as the steam pressure increases air is displaced down the drain. In a dynamic air-removal or prevacuum sterilizer, a vacuum pulls the air out before steam enters, creating a more efficient and rapid cycle time.[11] Flash sterilization is used for unwrapped cycles when items will be used immediately. There are also rigid containers specifically designed for flash cycles. Flash sterilized items require the same cleaning and decontamination as terminally sterilized items, and shortcuts cannot be taken or patient safety may be compromised.

There are different flash cycles depending on the particular items being flashed. Nonporous, metal items typically go into a 3-minute cycle and porous items or items with lumens require a 10-minute cycle. However, these parameters differ on whether a gravity or prevacuum cycle is being run, what temperature is selected, whether the load is wrapped or unwrapped, and may also vary with the type of rigid container purchased.[11] Manufacturer instructions for the rigid containers should be consulted before using them in flash cycles. Rigid containers also provide a safe method to transfer items from a sterilizer to the sterile field.[9] All flash cycles should be documented on a flow sheet in a consistent manner. Information required includes the patient name or medical record number, the operator of the sterilizer, cycle parameters, the item, date, and time, and reason for the cycle.[11]

The most important concern related to flash sterilization is the cleaning of the items prior to sterilization. Items to be flashed should be cleaned "according to the same standards as items intended for terminal sterilization."[9(p543)] Manufacturers' recommendations for many items include no instructions for sterilization in a flash cycle; these items should only be terminally sterilized. Other concerns related to flash sterilization involve the documentation of cycle and monitoring results, transport of the instruments by a method to decrease contamination, and a burn risk to staff and patients if the items are not properly cooled before use.[12]

Packaged items should be removed from the steam sterilizer and allowed to cool for 30 minutes up to 2 hours, depending on the size and configuration of the package.[5(p650)] The pressure within the package needs to equalize with the outside temperature or there is a risk of condensation within the pack being transferred through the package to the outside. Items should not be wrapped in blankets or towels for transport when they are too warm to touch. Any handling of these items compromises the sterility.

Ethylene oxide sterilization can be used for items that are sensitive to heat and/or moisture; this is a very effective low-temperature process.[6(p653–655)] All items, including lumens, are required to be completely dry before being packaged. The cycles require aeration before they can be used.

Low-temperature sterilization can also be achieved with hydrogen peroxide gas plasma. This process does not require aeration because the by-products are oxygen and water.[6(p655–656)] This process requires very specific lumen size regulations (length and diameter). The items must be completely dry before being placed into the chamber, to prevent cycle aborts. Many of the items processed via this method are sensitive to moisture and heat, and require hand washing. The rigid containers must be thoroughly dried before being placed in the chamber, in addition to the actual instruments themselves being dried. These items can be dried more rapidly in a commercial dryer, which can take an hour or more to adequately dry the items.

Ozone can also be used for terminal sterilization of heat- and moisture-sensitive items by oxidation. Cycles last 4 to 5 hours, and water and oxygen create the ozone in the system. The water should be deionized and the oxygen should be medical grade. No aeration is required. This inexpensive method of sterilization, while similar to low-temperature gas plasma sterilization, has some restrictions on lumen length and diameter.[13]

Vaporized hydrogen peroxide is the newest method of low-temperature sterilization available. This process works by "dropping liquid hydrogen peroxide onto a hot surface, instantaneously transforming it into a dry vapor form"[13(p43)] The peroxide needs a vacuum to be injected but the package penetration is very successful. Cycle time is about an hour, and it is less sensitive to moisture within packages. There are some restrictions on lumen length and diameter as with low-temperature gas plasma and ozone.

There should be a formal process in place within each organization to deal with loaner items.[6(p658–659)] Items should be received into sterile processing with an inventory list, at least 24 hours before the scheduled procedure, clean and in good working condition. Manufacturer instructions should be included and vendor representatives should be readily available to in-service operating room and sterile processing staff. These instruments are always considered contaminated on receipt and must arrive in time to be properly cleaned, packaged, and terminally sterilized. Many loaner trays are transported from facility to facility in the trunk of a vendor representative's car. Others are packaged for return to the original equipment manufacturer for inspection before release to another facility. However, because it is impossible to verify how instruments have been handled, cleaned, or inspected prior to receipt in the organization, it is imperative that all of these items be considered contaminated on arrival and not be handled with bare hands.[9]

When moisture is noticed after sterilized items are opened following terminal sterilization and cool-down, a wet pack should be automatically suspected. The moisture may be in droplet form that is visible, or there may be noticeable dampness. The moisture "can act as a wicking agent and can cause microorganisms to be drawn into the package, which compromises sterility."[9(p546)] The sterile processing department should be notified and a recall instituted for all items processed in the load.

Perioperative nurses should have a basic understanding of the various types of quality controls required for sterilized items, including mechanical controls such as graphs and printouts on sterilizers; chemical controls such as indicators and integrators, including autoclave tape, peel pouch dots, and rigid container arrows or breakaway locks; and biologic controls that are incubated and read in specific amounts of time. Whoever removes an item from a sterilizer is responsible for checking the cycle documentation to ensure parameters have been met. This check requires reviewing the printout or graph and ensuring the integrator has turned the appropriate color. Class 5 chemical indicator performance has been correlated with a biologic indicator and therefore can be used to release a load before the final biologic results are known.[9]

It is important to be able to look at a crinkled integrator from inside a sterile package, and to know when most likely the wrong integrator has been used for the sterilization process and the item cannot safely be used. Indicators measure only one parameter of sterilization, whereas integrators measure several parameters, making them more accurate. Some indicators change color after a period of time if they are placed into an autoclave and the sterilizer is never activated, or if they are left in a lighted area. Each organization should determine what types of indicators and integrators best serve their needs. One way to educate the sterile processing and operating room staff on the various indicators and integrators is to create handouts with tape and integrators both processed and unprocessed for each method of sterilization available in the organization.

EVENT-RELATED STERILITY

Sterility of the contents of a sterilized package is event related and depends on storage conditions, packaging materials, and handling.[14] "An event must occur to compromise package content sterility."[6(p641)] Temperature and humidity must be controlled where sterile goods are stored. Temperatures should not be greater than 24°C (75°F) and humidity should not be more than 70%. Air exchanges should be 4 per hour in a positive pressure room. There should be chemical indicators or integrators inside every package and chemical indicators on the outside of every package.[6(p642)] Internal indicators/integrators verify that air has been removed during the sterilization process and the sterilant has been able to penetrate to the center of the package. There should also be indicators or integrators on each level of a multilevel set.

Many events may compromise package sterility including:

- Multiple staff handling the packages
- Moisture from spills or placing items near sinks
- Airborne contaminants such as dust and lint
- Temperature or humidity problems, especially during the summer months
- Inadequate air exchanges
- Placement of sterile supplies in high traffic areas.

KEEPING OUTSIDE SHIPPING CONTAINERS IN THE STERILE STORAGE AREA

All sterile items should have the outside shipping containers removed in a breakdown area outside the sterile core.[6(p659–660)] Outside corrugated cardboard containers frequently contain bugs that may infiltrate a sterile stockroom if stored with unboxed sterile items that are processed both inside and outside the organization. Stock should also be rotated on a regular basis, using "first in, first out" technique,[6(p660)] and operating room staff should be instructed to restock and remove supplies based on this premise. Sterile items should be transported in enclosed carts when movement is outside the sterile core.

Product handling can lead to holes in outside wrappers of instrument packages. All wrapped items should have the wrapper checked for holes before placing items onto the sterile field. Holes can occur due to improper or rough handling, frequent handling, or quality issues. Occasional holes in a variety of items typically indicate a problem with handling the item, and it is difficult to determine where the improper handling might have occurred. Mishandling could happen during the processing or restocking phases, or when added to case carts in the sterile processing department. It could also occur in the operating room sterile storage room when items are restocked, or during handling in operating rooms themselves. These types of holes are difficult to predict. However, continuous holes in the wrappers of the same item indicate a quality issue that should be investigated further to be resolved. A different size of wrapper or changing to a rigid container typically can resolve these issues.

Holes also occur in peel pouch packages due to handling, and these packages should also be checked before use. Holding a pouch up to the light will most often alert the end user to a hole, but the package can also be checked after the scrub personnel have removed the instrument from the package. Therefore, it is important for scrub personnel not to return to their back table or handle other sterile products until the integrity of the outside package has been confirmed by the circulating nurse.

If construction or renovations are being considered within an operating room suite, it is imperative that containments installed be inspected by infection preventionists and operating room management to ensure they are adequate. Inadequate containments can compromise the integrity of sterile packages stored in the area and lead to the necessity to reprocess all items stored in the sterile room. This situation can cause shortages of priority instrumentation and the need to flash items for procedures in progress when the problem is identified.

ORIENTATION, EDUCATION, AND COMPETENCY

Orientations to perioperative nursing should include readings, videos, and hands-on training with sterilizers, biologic readers, integrators, and indicators. Nurses new to the perioperative setting should spend a week or two training on cleaning, decontamination, disinfection, and sterilization in the sterile processing department. This type of educational program provides the nurse with a true understanding of how the sterile processing department functions. It will assist the nurse in planning more accurately for patient care, allow operating room and sterile processing staff to get to know each other and to work side by side, and put faces and people behind the names thus creating a more congenial relationship between the two departments. If decontamination and sterilization are also done in the operating room suite, the new perioperative nurse should also spend time orienting to those areas and becoming familiar with the equipment they will be operating and the required documentation.

This orientation should be followed up with yearly competencies on high risk items that may be low in frequency of occurrence. The operating room manager or educator should work with the sterile processing manager to develop both the orientation program and the follow-up competencies. New products should be in-serviced with demonstrations and hands-on training that includes which items can be flash sterilized, how items are disassembled for cleaning, sterilization, and any other information critical to both end users.

Knowledge of regulatory requirements and best practices is important for nurses and managers of operating rooms in both hospitals and ambulatory surgical centers. A well-rounded orientation program followed with yearly competencies will provide nurses with the knowledge needed to safely perform cleaning, disinfection, and sterilization tasks. Clearly written policies and procedures will guide perioperative staff when performing tasks they do infrequently and with which they are therefore unfamiliar. Using the sterile processing department personnel as resources can also ensure that safe practices are followed. As patient advocates, perioperative nurses have many critical responsibilities. A foundation of knowledge related to sterile processing functions is essential to the well-rounded perioperative nurse.

Key Resources for Sterilization Decision-Making:
> AORN Recommended Practices
> AAMI ST79
> Manufacturer instructions on every device
> Spaulding's classification

Facilities Should Have Protocols for
> Managing loaner instruments/devices
> Education and training
> Competency verification
> Documentation of performance for each sterilizer load

Event-related sterility; rotation of stock/instrumentation

Key Points to Remember:

Five-day outdate on sterilized flexible endoscopes

Cleaning begins at point of use

Flash sterilization requires the same cleaning and decontamination as terminally sterilized items

Sets and individual instruments can take from 30 minutes to 2 hours to cool and cannot be handled before reaching room temperature

Recognition of various indicators and integrators, safe versus unsafe

Complex devices should completely disassembled for cleaning (refer to individual manufacturer instructions)

Separate sharps; open hinged instruments; don't put heavy instruments with delicate

Spray contaminated instruments with enzyme or soak in enzymatic or cover with wet towel before leaving the operating room

Peel pouches cannot be used within wrapped sets

Loaner instrumentation requires processing on-site; collaboration with vendors

Rotate stock and instruments on a daily basis.

REFERENCES

1. Association of Perioperative Registered Nurses. Perioperative standards and recommended practices. Recommended practices for cleaning, handling, and processing anesthesia equipment. Denver (CO): Association of Association of Perioperative Registered Nurses, Inc; 2009. p. 569–78.

2. Association of Perioperative Registered Nurses. Perioperative standards and recommended practices. Recommended practices for high-level disinfection. Denver (CO): Association of Association of Perioperative Registered Nurses, Inc; 2009. p. 579–94.

3. Association of Perioperative Registered Nurses. Perioperative standards and recommended practices. Recommended practices for cleaning and processing flexible endoscopes and endoscope accessories. Denver (CO): Association of Association of Perioperative Registered Nurses, Inc; 2009. p. 595–609.

4. Association of Perioperative Registered Nurses. Perioperative standards and recommended practices. Recommended practices for cleaning and care of surgical instruments and powered equipment. Denver (CO): Association of Association of Perioperative Registered Nurses, Inc; 2009. p. 611–35.

5. Association of Perioperative Registered Nurses. Perioperative standards and recommended practices. Recommended practices for selection and use of packaging systems for sterilization. Denver (CO): Association of Association of Perioperative Registered Nurses, Inc; 2009. p. 637–46.

6. Association of Perioperative Registered Nurses. Perioperative standards and recommended practices. Recommended practices for sterilization in the perioperative practice setting. Denver (CO): Association of Association of Perioperative Registered Nurses, Inc; 2009. p. 647–70.

7. Seavey R. The need for educated staff in sterile processing—patient safety depends on it. Perioperative Nursing Clinics 2009;4:181–92.

8. Meredith SJ, Sjorgen G. Decontamination: back to basics. J Perioper Pract 2008; 18(7):285–8.

9. Spry Cynthia. Understanding current steam sterilization recommendations and guidelines. AORN J 2008;88(4):537–50.
10. Hughes Chuck. Sterilization: would your facility pass a standards audit? AORN J 2008;87(1):176–82.
11. Moore Thomas K. "Chip". Today's sterilizer is not your father's water heater. AORN J 2009;90(1):81–8.
12. Carlo Arlene. The new era of flash sterilization. AORN J 2007;86(1):58–72.
13. Carter P, Wright M. The lowdown on low temperature sterilization for packaged devices. Healthcare Purchasing News July 2008;42–5.
14. Gilmour Diane. Instrument integrity and sterility: the perioperative practitioner's responsibilities. J Perioper Pract 2008;18(7):292–6.

High-Temperature Sterilization

Nyla "Skee" Japp, RN, PhD, CSPDM

KEYWORDS

• Sterilization • Surgical instruments
• Decontamination • Record keeping

Sterilization of instruments and devices is a complex process and cannot be managed by waving a magic wand. Improperly processed instruments and devices can be detrimental to patient safety—the device that is assumed to be safe for the patient may actually cause severe illness and even death. With that in mind, how does one ensure that the process of sterilizing surgical instruments and devices is effective? Success includes the education and effective participation of everyone who handles instruments from one point of use to the next, which includes the perioperative staff as well as those who work in the central sterile processing department (CSPD). Everyone handling surgical instruments affects the success of the sterilization process. Earlier, instruments were less complex and easier to manage; today we process a wide variety of instruments and devices, including powered devices, cameras and laparoscopic instrumentation, robotic instrumentation, and delicate microinstruments.

With patient safety a major concern and the increasing complexity of devices and instrumentation that are now being used for surgical procedures, infection preventionists should also participate in the education process and in routine monitoring of instrument and device sterilization. Visiting the CSPD only when a problem occurs or for an environmental safety audit is no longer appropriate. Today, the perioperative staff and the infection preventionist must participate actively in the sterilization process.

CLEANING, THE FIRST STEP TO STERILIZATION

The first step in the sterilization process is cleaning; sterilization cannot occur in the presence of bioburden. It is often said, "you can clean without sterilizing, but you cannot sterilize without cleaning."

Professional Central Sterile Processing Department Training and Mentoring, 13817 North 43rd Street, Phoenix, AZ 85032, USA
E-mail address: skeespdtraining@gmail.com

Perioperative Nursing Clinics 5 (2010) 273–280
doi:10.1016/j.cpen.2010.04.008
1556-7931/10/$ – see front matter © 2010 Elsevier Inc. All rights reserved.

periopnursing.theclinics.com

Cleaning is defined as the removal of contamination from an item to the extent necessary for further processing or for the intended use.[1] The Occupational Safety and Health Administration (OSHA)[2] defines decontamination as the use of physical or chemical means to remove, inactivate, or destroy blood-borne pathogens on a surface or item to the point where they are no longer capable of transmitting infectious particles and the surface or item is rendered safe for handling, use, or disposal. Although the items being cleaned vary from one facility to another, the fundamental principles of the cleaning and decontamination process remain the same. The first consideration is to request the cleaning and sterilization instructions from the original equipment manufacturer (OEM) for the device being cleaned. The OEM should provide detailed instructions, and the instructions should be followed in the decontamination area by all staff. The OEM instructions should always be kept in a notebook or file in the CSPD manager's office for reference.

Other considerations for the decontamination area include

- Design and location of the decontamination area
- Environmental design and controls
- Selection of cleaning products
- Water quality
- Staff knowledge of cleaning principles.

Cleaning can be accomplished either manually or mechanically. For delicate items, it is preferable to use a manual approach, which includes washing by hand and rinsing thoroughly. Items with lumens must be cleaned by inserting an appropriate-sized brush and brushing against the walls of the lumen in a back and forth movement. The cleaning brushes used during the day should also be decontaminated by running them through a cycle in the mechanical washer. Manual cleaning is also considered the method of choice for electrical and powered equipment that cannot be immersed in water, instrumentation that is complex in design, and as a preliminary step before mechanical washing to remove stubborn stains and soils. For effective manual cleaning, the water temperature should be between 109°F and 140°F (43°C–60°C) and should never exceed 140°F (60°C).[3] The final rinse should always be done with treated water to prevent mineral deposits. The pH of the cleaning solution should be between 7 and 9.

Mechanical decontamination involves washer-decontaminators, washer-sterilizers, ultrasonic cleaners, and cart washers. It is important never to overload the washer racks because the detergent and water will not reach each surface of the items being processed and thorough cleaning cannot be accomplished. It is always important to follow the manufacturer's guidelines when using any of the mechanical processes.

HIGH-TEMPERATURE STERILIZATION: SATURATED STEAM STERILIZATION

In the health care industry, steam sterilization has been recognized as the fastest and most economical method of sterilization. Steam sterilizers are available in a wide variety of sizes and configurations and offer different cycle selections.

The first recorded steam sterilizer resembled a pressure cooker. It was invented by Charles Chamberlain, a colleague of Louis Pasteur, in 1880. Steam sterilization requires pressurized steam at temperatures of 120°C and higher. Although today's sterilizers no longer resemble Chamberlain's, the technology of generating saturated steam is still relevant today.

The sterilizers are supplied with in-house steam normally coming from steam boilers located in the facilities services department or from self-contained packaged steam generators. Each system should be designed, monitored, and maintained to ensure that the quality, purity, and quantity of the steam are appropriate for effective sterile processing. Many issues can arise from the steam having to travel long distances to the sterilizers. It is important to ensure that the proper chemical amines are used in the boilers to help with the delivery of the steam.

Steam systems should be designed to ensure that a continuous and adequate supply of saturated steam is available to the sterilizer. The critical variables of steam quality are the dryness of the steam, expressed as a dryness fraction, and the level of noncondensable gas, expressed as a fraction of volume. Steam dryness should be between 97% and 100%, and the level of noncondensable gas should be such that it does not impair steam penetration into sterilization loads.[1] Steam that has less than 97% dryness results in wet packs in the sterilizer. Any wet pack is considered a sterilization failure and should not be considered a sterile tray. All trays and items that are in the wet load must be reprocessed starting with the decontamination process.

Tabletop Sterilizers

Small tabletop sterilizers are used most often in clinics and dental offices. These sterilizers generate their own steam from distilled or deionized water. Each day, before the sterilizer is used, it should be checked to ensure there is enough water in the reservoir for the number of loads to be processed.

Gravity Air Displacement Sterilizers

Gravity air displacement sterilizers are small to medium in size and are used in hospitals, outpatient clinics, sterile processing departments, and substerile rooms within the operating suite. The gravity sterilizer uses a passive air removal cycle that depends on gravity to remove all air from the sterilizer and from the items being sterilized. Sterilization cannot take place unless air is completely removed from the chamber of the sterilizer and the items being processed.

Liquids may be sterilized in a gravity displacement sterilizer because of the slow exhaust of the sterilizer. Cycle times differ, however, depending on the volume of liquid being sterilized. Biologic indicators should be run with the liquid cycle. The biologic vial should be suspended from a string in a container of the same solution being sterilized.

Dynamic Air Displacement Sterilizers

Dynamic air removal sterilizers, often referred to as prevacuum sterilizers, usually operate at temperatures higher than that of gravity sterilizers. Prevacuum sterilizers use an active air removal method by means of a vacuum pump that is equipped with the sterilizer. The higher temperature normally decreases the overall sterilization time of the cycle. When using a dynamic air removal system, one must always be sure that a Bowie-Dick test is done to ensure that there are no air leaks in the sterilizer. This test must be done on a daily basis in an empty chamber, and the results of the test documented in the sterilization records. The Bowie-Dick test must not be run with the biologic test pack. The purpose of the air removal test is to ensure that the vacuum pump on the sterilizer is functioning properly and that there are no air leaks in the chamber of the sterilizer. If air leaks are detected, the sterilizer should be placed out of service until a satisfactory air removal test is completed.

Liquids cannot be processed using a dynamic air removal sterilizer.

STEAM-FLUSH PRESSURE-PULSE STERILIZERS

Steam-flush pressure-pulse sterilizers use a repeated sequence of a steam flush and a pressure pulse to remove air from the sterilizer chamber and processed items. Similar to a prevacuum sterilizer, air is readily removed from the sterilizer chamber and items in the sterilizer. The difference is that the steam-flush pressure-pulse process is not susceptible to air leaks, making air removal tests unnecessary. Air removal occurs at a pressure higher than the atmospheric pressure, so no vacuum is required.

FLASH STERILIZERS

Flash sterilizers are often found in the operating room and in the labor and delivery and special procedure areas that perform invasive procedures. Flash sterilization should never be considered, except for emergency sterilization of instruments when there is no adequate time for terminal sterilization.

Flash sterilization normally has no packaging to impede air removal and steam penetration. Major issues associated with this sterilization process are not allowing enough time for proper and thorough cleaning of the device and transferring the sterilized device to the point of use without contaminating the item. Too often, flash sterilization is used because of inadequate inventory of instruments, which should be monitored by the facility, and where continuous flashing of a certain device or set is continually documented, additional sets should be purchased.

When flash containers are used, the manufacturer of the container must provide the facility with written instructions for cleaning, maintenance, and cycle exposure times.

MONITORING

Quality monitoring should include time, temperature, pressure, and moisture. Physical monitoring of the load provides real-time assessment that the sterilization parameters were achieved during the cycle. Physical monitors include time, temperature, and pressure recorders, such as charts displays, digital printouts, and gauge readings. The physical monitors should be reviewed for correct conditions, and the review should be documented by initialing and dating the printout. These physical monitors should be checked for functionality before the beginning of the cycle, the cycle conditions verified by reading, and the printout marked by the operator at the end of the cycle for correct cycle information and saved as part of record keeping. Sterilizers without recording devices should not be used.[1]

If physical monitoring shows a sterilizer malfunction or suspicious operation that cannot be corrected immediately, the cycle should be terminated and the load considered unsterile. The sterilizer should be removed from service, and the malfunction corrected. Before reusing the sterilizer, biologic testing should be done to ensure that the problem has been identified and corrected. The results of the biologic testing should be documented.

Packaging errors can interfere with steam sterilization because these monitors only measure the chamber temperature and not the temperature inside the package. For this reason, chemical and biologic indicators must be included to the department quality-monitoring program.

For tabletop sterilizers that do not have a dynamic air removal system, Bowie-Dick testing is not needed. For tabletop sterilizers that do have a dynamic air removal system, the Bowie-Dick test is needed to ensure that there are no air leaks in the sterilizer. The Bowie-Dick test should be run on an empty chamber by itself, and the results of the test documented in the daily sterilization results.

HIGH-TEMPERATURE STERILIZATION: DRY HEAT STERILIZATION

Dry heat sterilization requires high temperature and a lengthy time cycle. Sterilization is accomplished by conduction, as heat is absorbed by an item's exterior surface and passed inward to the next layer. Eventually, the entire item reaches the proper temperature needed for sterilization. The process by which dry heat sterilization kills microorganisms is called oxidation, which is literally the burning up of all forms of viable life on the item.

One advantage of dry heat sterilization is the ability to sterilize powders, oils, petroleum-based items, and unassembled needles and syringes. Dry heat sterilization is not widely used in health care facilities in the United States because of the high temperatures and long exposure times required for sterilization. Some hospitals, however, use dry heat sterilization to sterilize talcum powder used in some specialized thoracic surgical procedures.

The required parameters for dry heat sterilization are temperature and time. The temperature required is between 320°F and 338°F (160°C–170°C), and time, a 2- to 4-hour cycle.[3] The specific exposure time and temperature depend on the type of sterilizer; therefore, it is imperative that the manufacturer's recommendations for exposure time and temperature be followed for the items being processed.

Packaging materials used for dry heat sterilization include heat-resistant glass (eg, Petri dishes, test tubes, and small jars), stainless steel trays, aluminum foil, nylon films, and cotton muslin (minimum 400 thread count), if the chamber does not exceed 400°F (240°C).[4] Dry heat cannot be used with rubber and fabrics of lesser thread count, as the materials will deteriorate during the sterilization cycle.

There are 2 types of dry heat sterilizers:

1. Gravity convection sterilizer. This sterilizer depends on gravity to lower the heat from the top to the bottom. As air within the chamber is heated, it rises and displaces cooler air that descends into the lower part of the chamber. This circulation pattern causes inconsistent temperatures within the chamber, making it the less-preferred method because dry heat sterilization requires that a given temperature be reached and maintained for a specific period. When patterns are inconsistent, it makes it difficult to monitor the sterilization process in a gravity sterilizer.
2. Mechanical convection sterilizer. This sterilizer contains a blower that actively forces heated air throughout all areas of the sterilizer chamber. This flow creates a uniform temperature, and the equal transfer of heat throughout the load, making this process the easier method to monitor. With this advantage, the mechanical convection type sterilizer is the preferred sterilizer in many facilities using dry heat sterilization.

Biologic monitoring of the sterilization process should be done at least weekly, and the results of the monitoring documented. The construction and placement of the biologic monitor should be in accordance with the sterilizer manufacturer's written recommendations. The spore used for dry heat sterilization is *Bacillus atrophaeus*. Conventional biologic indicators in plastic vials cannot be used because of the increased temperatures. A spore strip placed in a glassine envelope is the appropriate method used for monitoring the sterilization cycle. Only biologic and chemical indicators that have been validated for dry heat cycles should be used.

HIGH-TEMPERATURE STERILIZATION: WASHER-STERILIZERS

Washer-sterilizers are often found in the sterile processing decontamination area, clinics, and surgery centers. They are capable of washing and sterilizing the instruments. Washer-sterilizers are mostly used for decontaminating instruments before cleaning. This process does not provide a terminal sterilization cycle for immediate patient use. All items processed in a washer-sterilizer must still be cleaned and sterilized using either a terminal process or a flash sterilization process.

Regardless of the steam sterilization method used, one should always be sure that all requirements for steam sterilization have been met. These requirements include:

- Contact: The most frequent reason for sterilization failure is the lack of contact between steam and the microorganisms on the entire surface of the device being sterilized. Contact failures occur mainly because the device or items have not been properly cleaned. Steam cannot penetrate protein soils that have been left on the device from not thoroughly cleaning the item. Other reasons for failure may include packages being wrapped too tightly, items not being properly positioned on the sterilization cart, the drain on the sterilizer not being cleaned, or other mechanical malfunctions.
- Temperature: Steam sterilization requires specific temperatures to achieve sterilization. The most common temperatures used today include 250°F (121°C) and between 270°F and 275°F (132.2°C–134°C).
- Time: Time is required for bacteria to be killed and sterilization to be accomplished. Today, more than ever before, manufacturing guidelines must be obtained and followed for specific sterilization times. Many manufacturers require extended cycle times depending on the device being sterilized. Be certain that a list of guidelines is available for all staff to follow. These times should be posted by the steam sterilizers in an area that is easily seen by all the staff.
- Moisture: Dry saturated steam is required to achieve sterilization of all devices. This steam should have between 97% to 100% dryness.

SPECIAL CONSIDERATIONS FOR CREUTZFELDT-JAKOB DISEASE

All known instances of iatrogenic Creutzfeldt-Jakob disease (CJD) have resulted from exposure to infectious brain, pituitary, or eye tissue. Transmissibility is directly related to the concentration of prions in the tissues.

Because it is difficult to inactivate prions, the causative agent of CJD, special procedures are used to process instruments that have been used on a patient with known or suspected CJD. A system must be in place at all facilities for identifying instruments that are potentially exposed to an infected patient with CJD. This system must be known by all of the operating room as well as central sterile processing personnel.

Processing devices contaminated with high-risk tissue, defined as brain, including dura mater, spinal cord, and eye tissue, from high-risk patients (known or suspected of having CJD).

1. Devices that are constructed such that cleaning procedures result in effective tissue removal (surgical instruments) can be cleaned and then sterilized at 134°C for 18 minutes or more in a prevacuum sterilizer or at 121°C to 132°C for 60 minutes in a gravity displacement sterilizer. Routine decontamination and sterilization processes follow this procedure.
2. Devices that are impossible or difficult to clean should be discarded.
3. Flash sterilization should *not* be used for reprocessing these devices.

Processing devices contaminated with low-risk tissue, defined as cerebrospinal fluid, kidney, liver, spleen, lung, and lymph node tissue from high-risk patients.

1. Devices can be cleaned and disinfected or sterilized using conventional methods of high-level disinfection, thermal sterilization, or chemical sterilization.
2. Environmental surfaces contaminated with low-risk tissues require only standard disinfection using disinfectants recommended by OSHA for decontaminating blood-contaminated surfaces.

Processing devices contaminated with no-risk tissue, defined as peripheral nerve tissue, intestinal tissue, bone marrow, blood, leukocytes, serum, thyroid gland tissue, adrenal gland tissue, heart tissue, skeletal muscle, adipose tissue, gingival tissue, prostate tissue, testicular tissue, placental tissue, tears, nasal mucus, saliva, sputum, urine, feces, semen, vaginal secretions, and breast milk from high-risk patients.

1. Devices can be cleaned and disinfected or sterilized using conventional methods for high-level disinfection, thermal sterilization, or chemical sterilization.
2. Endoscopes (except for neurosurgical endoscopes) are likely to be contaminated only with no-risk materials; therefore, standard cleaning and high-level disinfection protocols are adequate for reprocessing.
3. Environmental surfaces contaminated with no-risk tissues or fluids require only standard disinfection using disinfectants recommended by OSHA for decontaminating blood-contaminated surfaces.

PREVENTIVE MAINTENANCE PROGRAMS

All autoclaves, washer-decontaminators, sonic cleaners, heat-sealers, and irrigators should be routinely maintained in the sterile processing department. A preventive maintenance program allows equipment to be maintained in proper operating condition by providing planned inspections and by detecting and correcting failures before they occur.

RECORD KEEPING

Record keeping documents what items have been processed and provides monitoring control evidence for those items. Record keeping is an absolute necessity for any facility involved in sterilization of surgical instrumentation and materials for disbursement. In the event of a recall, there must be a system in place to enable finding and reprocessing items that are in question. This is accomplished by keeping accurate records of every item processed.

Each item processed should be labeled with a lot control number to enable retrieval of items in the event of a recall, to trace problems such as wet packs to their source, and to facilitate proper stock rotation. This number also enables traceability for items reprocessed to the patient as well as for implantable devices. The control number should include the sterilizer number, the date of sterilization, and the cycle number.

An expiration date or statement that the contents are sterile unless package is damaged or opened should be affixed to each item for proper stock rotation. Each item should be inspected and not used if damaged or opened.

Sterilization data should be recorded and maintained for each load to ensure real-time monitoring of the process, to ensure that cycle parameters were met, and to assist with recalls and establish accountability.[1] The information for each sterilization cycle should include

- Lot number
- Contents of the load
- Exposure time and temperature if not on a recording chart
- Operator identification

- Results of biologic testing
- Results of the Bowie-Dick testing
- Results of chemical indicator (CI) in the process challenge device
- Any reports of inconclusive or nonresponsive CIs in the load.

Sterilizer records should be retained according to the policy and procedure established by the individual health care facility.

When a positive biologic indicator is obtained, the infection control department should be notified immediately. This notification should be followed by a written report. If it is determined that the sterilization failure was not the result of operator error, items processed in that sterilizer since the last negative biologic indicator results should be considered unsterile. They should be retrieved, if possible, and reprocessed. The sterilizer in question should be taken out of service.

Most frequently, failures are caused by human errors as opposed to mechanical failures. When human error is identified, in addition to the possibility of the need for additional training, assessment of the situation should include opportunities for environmental engineering, changes in process or the physical environment, that might decrease the likelihood of human error.

Monitoring the sterilization process is a complex and important function for health care sterile processing departments. Complete and accurate records are of utmost importance. Documentation assures the monitoring of the sterilization process, assures that cycle parameters have been met, and establishes accountability.

SUMMARY

Health care facilities are requiring that we optimize our processes without sacrificing our quality. They want it done the right way the first time. The "good old days" and the "way we always did it" are no longer acceptable rationale. Today we must effectively team up with infection preventionists, perioperative nurses, and physicians to explore effective approaches to ensuring patient safety. We must implement proper training and education of all individuals involved in the handling of sterile instruments and devices; perioperative nurses who understand the principles and practice of sterilization can participate effectively in ensuring the sterility of the items used in the operating room. Infection preventionists can be advocates for sterile processing by stressing the importance of what we do and how we do it in delivering safe patient care. It is important to have written policies and procedures; however, they must be followed to be of value. Surgical site infections can be reduced by ensuring proper cleaning, packaging, and sterilization of instruments. In addition, the cost of health care would be reduced by savings millions spent on hospital-associated infections.

REFERENCES

1. The Association for the Advancement of Medical Instrumentation. Comprehensive guide to steam sterilization and sterility assurance in health care facilities. ST79. Arlington (VA): ANSI/AAMI; 2006.
2. Occupational Safety and Health Administration. Occupational exposure to blood borne pathogens. 21 CFR 1910.1030.
3. Sterile Processing University, LLC. The basics of sterile processing. 3rd edition. Lebanon (NJ): 2007.
4. Central Service Training Manual. International Association for Central Service and Materials Management. Chicago (IL): 2007.

Low-Temperature Sterilization: Are You In the Know?

Cheri Ackert-Burr, RN, MSN, CNOR

KEYWORDS
- Hydrogen peroxide sterilization • Ozone sterilization
- Paracetic acid sterilization • Ethylene oxide sterilization

Today's perioperative nurse is expected to do more with less, be knowledgeable about patient and surgical team safety issues, stay current with recommended practices, and operate within a budget. Not only must nurses deliver high-quality patient care, but they must continuously seek ways to reduce operating costs. Low-temperature sterilization provides an opportunity to deliver safe patient care at a reasonable cost.

HISTORY OF LOW-TEMPERATURE STERILIZATION

Historically, most surgical instruments were processed using steam or dry heat. Over time and with improved technology, surgical procedures became more sophisticated and the associated medical devices become more complex. Much of the new instrumentation was sensitive to heat and moisture, requiring an alternative to steam sterilization. Low-temperature sterilization with ethylene oxide (EtO), a very effective microbiocidal chemical agent, was introduced in the early 1950s (Occupational Safety and Health Administration [OSHA], 2009).[1] No other options were available until paracetic acid was introduced in 1988.[2,3] Instruments processed in paracetic acid must be used immediately, this introducing the term "just-in-time processing."

Hydrogen peroxide gas plasma technology has been available since 1993,[2,4] with ozone sterilization technology becoming available in 2003.[2,5] The latest technology to be cleared by the Food and Drug Administration (FDA) in 2007 was vaporized hydrogen peroxide gas.[2,3] All sterilizers used for sterilizing surgical instruments are considered Class II medical devices and must follow specific guidelines for manufacturing and submission to the FDA before being marketed for sale.[2,6]

TSO3 – Department, Education, University of Texas at Arlington, College of Nursing, 701 South Neederman Drive, Arlington, TX 76019, USA
E-mail address: cackert-burr@hotmail.com

Perioperative Nursing Clinics 5 (2010) 281–290
doi:10.1016/j.cpen.2010.05.002
1556-7931/10/$ – see front matter © 2010 Published by Elsevier Inc.
periopnursing.theclinics.com

SAFETY

To Err is Human, published in 1999 by the Institute of Medicine,[7] stimulated the focus of the entire health care delivery system on patient safety. Surgical site infections are considered "never events." In 2003, the Joint Commission on Accreditation of Healthcare Organizations (JCAHO) and the Centers for Medicare and Medicaid Services (CMS) jointly produced the Surgical Care Improvement Project (SCIP),[8] which identified core measures to improve surgical site infection rates. Data collected based on the implementation of SCIP measures demonstrated improvement in preventing surgical site infections. More recently, CMS implemented nonpayment for adverse events and conditions "not present on admission."

As a patient advocate and team leader during a surgical procedure, the perioperative nurse is responsible for monitoring all aspects of aseptic technique. This includes monitoring to ensure the sterility of instruments and devices before they are placed on a sterile field. The integrity of sterile packages must be checked before opening, and indicators on the outside and inside of sterile packages must indicate that the items are sterile.

Sterilization of surgical instruments is a team process that incorporates a system of checks and balances. Everyone who handles instruments from point of use to terminal sterilization must collaborate to ensure that all of the steps in the process of producing sterile instruments and supplies are addressed properly. Sterile processing department (SPD) decontaminates, cleans, and checks each item, assembles instrument sets, and processes the instruments with one of the hospital's available sterilization technologies.[4,9,10] SPD technicians monitor the process of sterilization with mechanical, biologic, and chemical indicators/integrators that visually tell the technician that the instruments have completed the sterilization process.[11] The technician then signs the documents, records the results, and transports the instruments to a sterile storage area.

In the operating room, where the sterile instruments, medical devices, or supplies are used, the perioperative nurse verifies sterility by inspecting package integrity and checking external and internal indicators as supplies are opened. It is critical for nurses to have a working knowledge of currently available low-temperature sterilization technologies as they determine which items have been correctly processed or have not been processed before they are used for the surgical procedure.[12-15] During the procedure, the scrub person keeps the instruments as clean as possible, then prepares them for transport to SPD, separating them appropriately and ensuring that blood and bioburden do not dry on the instruments, which would make it very difficult to clean them and process them for resterilization. The scrub person must also indicate when an instrument needs repair, eg, scissors that are not sharp enough or a fiberoptic cord that no longer carries sufficient light. The condition in which SPD receives instruments from the operating room (OR) (eg, sets intact, moistened to prevent bioburden from drying, defective instruments identified) affects their ability to prepare them properly for future use **Fig. 1**.

Every sterilizer must meet the Sterility Assurance Level (SAL) of 10^{-6} or a 12-log reduction of microbial bioburden.[2,16-19] With each log reduction, 90% of all microbes are killed; a 6-log reduction ensures that 99.999% of microbes are killed. Each spore strip used in the biologic testing of sterilizers is inoculated with 1 million nonpathogenic spore-producing bacteria. Low-temperature sterilizers use *Geobacillus stearothermophilus* and/or *Bacillus atrophaeus*.

The sterilizers must also be tested for a wide range of material compatibility and lumen claims. Medical device manufacturers will choose to test their instruments in one or more of the available sterilization technologies. When nurses consider

Sterilization in Hospitals

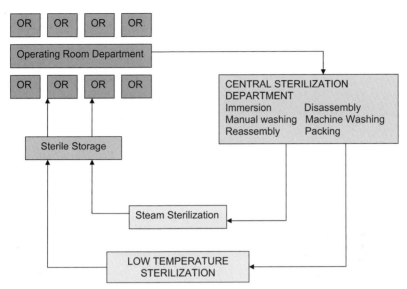

Fig. 1. Sterilization in hospitals.

purchasing medical devices, part of the decision depends on the device manufacturer's recommendations for sterilization processing. To make appropriate decisions, nurses must be aware of the advantages and disadvantages of the technologies being considered (**Table 1**).

LOW-TEMPERATURE STERILIZATION TECHNOLOGIES

EtO has been used the longest for low-temperature sterilization and is considered to have very effective microbiocidal properties. This very effective technology, however, offers many challenges for the user; it is the most regulated sterilization technology in use today. EtO is an odorless, colorless gas that can be toxic if handled improperly. OSHA exposure limits for EtO are 1 ppm (parts per million) over a time weight average (TWA) of 8 hours or 5 ppm excursion limit. EtO is considered to be a carcinogen, is mutagenic, and can produce neurotoxicity and sensitization. Most exposure incidences occur during inadequate aeration procedures (OSHA, 2009).[1] To avoid numerous safety concerns, EtO must be used only as recommended by OSHA.

Federal and state regulations from OSHA, FDA, and the Environmental Protection Agency (EPA) must be followed for the safe installation, continued use, and monitoring of EtO. Medical records of employees working with EtO are to be kept on file for 30 years after the employee terminates working at the facility. The sterilization guidelines for using EtO as a sterilant fall under the American National Standards Institute/Association for the Advancement of Medical Instrumentation (ANSI/AAMI) ST 41:2008 Guidelines.[17]

Mechanical monitoring for incidental exposure is mandatory for the facility. Monitors are required that will sound an alarm when an EtO leak occurs. EtO sterilizers are usually installed in negative-pressure rooms with a contained ventilation system venting to the outside. The current EtO machines have safety features that keep the machine in a locked position until specially trained personnel can determine the problem and how to fix it. Medical devices and supplies in the load will remain in the locked chamber

Table 1
Advantages and disadvantages of current low temperature sterilization technologies

Sterilization Process	Advantages	Disadvantages
Ethylene oxide (EtO) 100% and mixed gas	Compatible with most medical materials Penetrates packaging materials and device lumens Single-dose cartridge and negative-pressure chamber (minimizes the potential for gas leak and EtO exposure) 100% Cycle is easy to control and monitor All packaging materials are usable 35°C–55°C (95°F–131°F)	Cycle time is 8–12 hours Aeration is required EtO is a carcinogen, mutagenic, and flammable EtO emissions are regulated by states, but can be put through a catalytic convertor to make emissions safer Must be mechanically monitored Employee health records must be saved for 30 years after last employment date Complicated installation process
Paracetic acid	Cycle time 30–45 min Environmentally friendly by-products Sterilant flows through endoscope, which facilitates salt, protein, and microbe removal 50°C–55°C (122°F–132.8°F)	Point-of-use system, must be used within 2 hours of processing Biologic monitoring may not be suitable for routine monitoring Can process only heat-sensitive items Limited number of items processed at one time Sterilant needs to be refrigerated
Hydrogen peroxide gas plasma	Cycle time 45–75 minutes Equipment is simple to operate Equipment requires only an electrical outlet for installation Compatible with wide range of materials No toxic residues on instrument at completion of cycle 45°C–55°C (113°F–131°F)	Cellulose (paper), linens, and liquids cannot be processed Chamber size varies, some are smaller, may require more loads Limited lumen claims Requires specialty packaging (polypropylene wrap, polyolefin pouches, and special container trays)
Hydrogen peroxide gas vapor	Cycle time 55 minutes Equipment is simple to operate Equipment requires only an electrical outlet for installation Compatible with wide range of materials No toxic residues on instrument at completion of cycle 45°C–50°C (113°F–122°F)	Cellulose (paper), linens, and liquids cannot be processed Chamber size varies, some are smaller, may require more loads Limited lumen claims Requires specialty packaging (polypropylene wrap, polyolefin pouches, and special container trays)
Ozone	Equipment is simple to operate Has best lumen claims of new low-temperature sterilization technologies Requires electrical plug and medical-grade oxygen source for installation No toxic residues after processing or with a cancelled cycle No sterilant to handle Containers can be stacked 30°C–36°C (86°F–97°F)	Cycle time is 4.5 hours Medical-grade oxygen source required for installation Medical device testing by manufacturers still ongoing

All sterilization processes demonstrated Sterility Assurance Level 10^{-6} before being cleared by the Food and Drug Administration.
Data from Refs. [3,14]; TSO$_3$, 2008.

until the aeration cycle has been completed or manually removed and aerated in a safe environment room. This practice minimizes the potential exposure to EtO.

EtO uses a variety of packaging materials as recommended by the sterilizer manufacturer. Paper/Mylar or Tyvek/Mylar pouches may be used as well as recommended fabric wrappers, medical crepe paper wraps, polypropylene wraps, and numerous types of self-contained containers. Several companies make chemical indicators/integrators for use in EtO. Each manufacturer's instructions should be followed when interpreting the color or indicator change after processing. The biologic used for EtO is *Geobacillus subtilis.* EtO kills by alkylation, causing the microorganism to be unable to metabolize or reproduce, resulting in death.[2,20] The most difficult constraint to using EtO is the 12- to 16-hour processing time, which can be an important consideration when you are looking at inventory levels of expensive equipment and the number of like items that will be needed to process those items in EtO.

OXIDATIVE TECHNOLOGIES

The more recent low-temperature sterilization technologies cleared by the FDA are considered oxidative processes. Oxidating agents are highly reactive. Oxidation is the loss of an electron by a molecule, atom, or ion. Oxidizing agents will contribute oxygen, extract hydrogen, or extract electrons in a reaction.[21] Oxidation is normally thought of as a process that causes burning or a situation where rust is the result of a chemical change. Low-temperature technologies reduce the potential for instrument damage significantly.

Two types of surgical stainless steel instruments are used in surgery. Martensitic or 400-grade steel provides hard steel that holds a prolonged sharp edge, especially important for orthopedic instruments and other instruments used on bone. Austenitic steel or 300-grade steel is also considered stainless steel, but is more malleable and used where flexible instruments are needed. Both types of stainless steel will rust if not cared for properly during processing.

The 3 oxidative low-temperature sterilization processes used in the health care industry today are ozone, paracetic acid, and vaporized hydrogen peroxide gas and hydrogen peroxide gas plasma. Each oxidative process causes a different chemical reaction, usually leading to the destruction of the cell membrane and causing death of any organic organism.[12] *Geobacillus stearothermophilus* is the biologic organism used to challenge all of these sterilization processes.

Each technology offers advantages as well as challenges for processing medical devices and surgical instruments (see **Table 1**). **Table 2** offers operating cost comparisons and what it would cost to use each technology at the same level or capacity. **Table 3** lists patient and staff safety considerations for all low-temperature sterilization technologies. **Fig. 2** provides a comparison for lumen claims for the ozone and hydrogen peroxide technologies. These tables and the figure may be used as resources for making purchasing decisions among complementary technologies to determine the best fit for a facility's specific sterile processing needs.

PARACETIC ACID

The disinfection and sterilization properties of paracetic acid have been recognized for more than 100 years. Paracetic acid has been used as a sterilant in hospital settings since 1985.[2] Paracetic acid is acetic acid, vinegar with an extra oxygen atom in an equilibrium equation.[21] The extra oxygen atom of paracetic acid is extremely reactive with most cellular components, causing cell death. Buffers and anticorrosives are added to the paracetic acid, making it a very effective disinfectant or sterilizing agent.

Table 2
Yearly sterilant operating cost per low-temperature sterilization process

Low-Temperature Sterilization Technologies

300 Days	EtO Mixed Gas	100% EtO 5 XL	HP Plasma STERRAD NX	HP Plasma STERRAD 100S/NX	HP Plasma STERRAD 200	Vaporized HP V-Pro 1	Ozone Sterizone 125L
Useable (measured) Capacity (cu. ft.) per sterilization cycle	1.5	4.8	1.0	1.7	3.2	1.7	3.8
Sterilization loads/day[a]	1	1 load in 3 sterilizers	14	9	5	9	4
Average sterilant cost/cycle[b]	$175.00	$10.00	$12.00	$12.00	$25.00	$10.00	$1.00
Average sterilant cost/day	$175.00	$30.00	$168.00	$108.00	$125.00	$90.00	$4.00
Annual sterilant cost	$52,000	$9000	$50,400	$32,500	$37,500	$27,000	$1200 Formula for sterilant cost: Loads per day × cost per cycle × 300 days = cost.

Abbreviations: cu ft, cubic feet; EtO, ethylene oxide; HP, hydrogen peroxide.
[a] Equal capacity and throughput of medical devices.
[b] Costs are approximate; price will vary according to the facility's group purchasing organization (GPO) and contract pricing.
Data from Refs. [3,14]; TSO_3, 2008.

Table 3
Safety considerations for low-temperature sterilization technologies

Sterilization Process	Safety Considerations
Ethylene oxide (EtO)	State and federal regulations are very stringent Mandatory mechanical monitoring Canisters must be stored in a flammable liquid storage container Machine must be stored in a negative-pressure room Rebreathing apparatus must be worn if H tanks need to be changed or if there is a leak Incomplete aeration could result in patient exposure to toxic residues leading to respiratory distress
Paracetic acid	Personal protective equipment, for handling disposal of canisters
Hydrogen peroxide gas plasma	Personal protective equipment, for handling items with canceled cycle Personal protective equipment when disposing of cassette box
Hydrogen peroxide gas vapor	Personal protective equipment when disposing of canisters
Ozone	None

Data from American National Standard Institute/Association for the Advancement of Medical Instrumentation. *ST58:2005, Chemical sterilization and high-level disinfection in health care facilities.* Arlington, VA: Association for the Advancement of Medical Instrumentation; 2006.

The sterilization process takes approximately 30 to 45 minutes depending on water pressure and temperature.[2] Nurses and technicians responsible for sterilizing reusable medical devices with paracetic acid need to have completed the manufacturer-required skills training.

The instruments processed in paracetic acid must be moisture tolerant, but may be heat sensitive. Certain medical devices require connectors that allow the liquid sterilant, under pressure, to pass through the lumens of the devices. Paracetic acid used in health care settings is a liquid process and is recognized as a "just-in-time" process. The sterilized items remain in the sterilizer and must be used within 2 hours after processing; they cannot be removed, packaged, and stored. Items targeted for paracetic acid processing include flexible endoscopes, rigid endoscopes, light cords, and cameras. The nurse may find this process appropriate for other medical devices, but must follow the medical device and the sterilizer manufacturer's recommendations for processing. The FDA has cleared a newer model of the Steris System1E but has placed specific processing recommendations for medical devices, clearly designating some as high-level disinfections and some for sterilization processing. The nurse or technician will need to contact the manufacturer for itemized processing instructions.

HYDROGEN PEROXIDE GAS PLASMA AND HYDROGEN PEROXIDE VAPOR

Hydrogen peroxide (H_2O_2) gas plasma and vaporized hydrogen peroxide are also very effective oxidizing agents. Both use a 59% hydrogen peroxide solution for the sterilization cycle. Vaporized hydrogen peroxide has been used to disinfect papers, buildings, and material exposed to anthrax.[21] H_2O_2 produces hydroxyl radicals that interrupt the cell membrane of organic matter, effectively killing the cell (Russell and colleagues 2001).[12]

Hydrogen peroxide gas plasma was cleared for the health care market by the FDA in 1993, whereas vaporized hydrogen peroxide was cleared in the fall of 2007.[1–3] It is compatible with a wide range of materials. The cycle times for the sterilization process

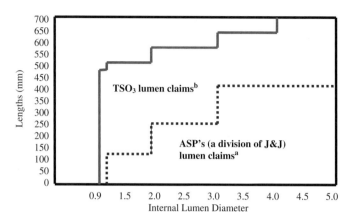

Ozone and Hydrogen Peroxide Plasma and Vapor Lumen Claims
[a]Hydrogen peroxide plasma and vapor can process a maximum of 20 lumens
[b]Ozone has no maximum lumen number limitation

Internal diameter	Length	Inches
≥ 0.9 mm	≤ 485 mm	19.09
≥ 1 mm	≤ 500 mm	19.69
≥ 2 mm	≤ 575 mm	21.64
≥ 3 mm	≤ 650 mm	25.59
≥ 4 mm	≤ 700 mm	27.56

Fig. 2. TSO_3 and ASP's FDA-cleared lumen claims for sterilization. *Data from* Advanced Sterilization Products, product documentation. (n.d.). Available at: http://www.aspjj.com/Products. Accessed June 9, 2009; TSO_3, 2008.

can vary from 35 minutes to 75 minutes. Different machines have different cycle times and different capabilities for processing surgical instruments. Choosing the correct cycle can present a challenge for nurses, as they must know the recommendations for different instruments and what medical devices are compatible with the H_2O_2 process as well as the lumen limitations of each machine. Each model has different limitations for number of lumens and has different lumen size restrictions. Lumen limitations are listed in **Fig. 2**.

The hydrogen peroxide sterilization process is environmentally friendly, as the by-products are oxygen and vaporized water; however, safety precautions recommend the nurse wear gloves when handling items from a cancelled load or when changing the cassette collection box. There are some materials that are incompatible with H_2O_2 processing; these include cellulose material, liquids, linen, and paper. Packaging required for this system is polypropylene wrap, Tyvek/Mylar peel pouches, and special rigid containers recommended by the sterilizer manufacturer.

Medical device manufacturers and sterilizer manufacturers provide the most current recommendations for instrument processing in H_2O_2 systems. Hydrogen peroxide sterilization can meet the fast turnaround times required for a busy surgical schedule, but it is considered more expensive to operate on a per-cycle basis than other low-temperature processes (see **Table 2**).

OZONE

Ozone has been used since 1840 for food preservation, and since 1870 for blood purification. Ozone is used in industry for water reclamation, deodorization, food preservation, water treatment, and as an alternative therapy for some disease processes.

The ozone sterilization technology was cleared by the FDA for market in 2003 (TSO_3, 2008).[2,5,22] Ozone is highly effective as an oxidizing agent for low-temperature sterilization. Ozone uses medical-grade oxygen as the source chemical and electricity as the force to generate ozone in a deep vacuum within the sterilization chamber. Ozone sterilizes by producing a free oxygen atom that oxidizes proteins and enzymes of any organic matter, causing the death of the organism (TSO_3, 2008).

The first-generation ozone sterilizer has a 4.5-hour cycle time, but is compatible with most heat- and moisture-sensitive instruments and can sterilize most materials, except cellulosics, liquids, and latex items . There are no restrictions on the number of lumened instruments that can be placed in one sterilizer load. Lumen size restrictions are addressed in the manufacturer's recommendations. The next-generation of ozone sterilizers (based on FDA clearance) will combine ozone with hydrogen peroxide to produce cycle times ranging from 46 minutes to 100 minutes, comparable with other low-temperature sterilization technologies.

Safety is an important feature of ozone sterilization, as the by-products of the process are oxygen and humidified air. The sterilant is generated using piped-in oxygen and electricity; there is no sterilant container to handle when starting or completing a cycle. At the completion of each process a ventilation phase converts any residual ozone into oxygen and humidified air. There are no toxic residues to harm either staff or patient.

The manufacturer of the ozone sterilizer recommends specific wraps, paper peel pouches, and anodized aluminum containers for packaging of items to be processed. The ozone sterilization process has the most economical operating costs of any of the low-temperature sterilization processes and the most extensive lumen claims (see **Table 2**).[23]

SUMMARY

Advances in surgical technology result in more complex instruments as well as new sterilization processes to manage them. The process of sterilizing surgical instruments and medical devices is complex and requires that perioperative nurses consistently update their knowledge of the various sterilization processes, regulatory standards, manufacturers' recommendations, and changing standards of practices. Every low-temperature sterilization process has its own set of parameters and chemical indicators for determining accurate processing procedures. The more low-temperature processes used, the more opportunity for confusion with processing.

Providing sterile instruments, supplies, and medical devices for surgery requires the collaboration of perioperative nurses and SPD personnel. Each individual must accept the responsibility for participating in the process, communicating effectively, and sharing knowledge to provide safe patient care.

REFERENCES

1. Occupational Health and Safety Administration (OSHA) United States Department of Labor. Regulatory review of the occupational safety and health administrations' ethylene oxide standard [29 CFR 1910.1047]. Available at: http://www.osha.gov/dea/lookback/ethylene_oxide-lookback.html; 2009. Accessed June 9, 2009.
2. Food & Drug Administration. Low temperature sterilization methods. Available at: www.fda.gov; 2009. Accessed June 9, 2009.
3. Steris Corporation products documents. Available at: http://www.steris.com/healthcare/sterile.cfm. Accessed June 9, 2009.
4. Advanced Sterilization Products, products documentation. Available at: http://www.aspjj.com/Products. Accessed June 9, 2009.

5. TSO$_3$ Operator's Manual. Sterizone®125L Sterilizer. Quebec City: TSO$_3$, Inc; 2008. Ontario, Canada.

6. Becker B. FDA, 510(k)s, and standards. Healthcare Purchasing News Online. Available at: www.hpnonline.com; 2008. Accessed June 9, 2009.

7. Kohn LT, Corrigan JM, Donaldson MS, editors. Committee on Quality of Health Care in America, Institute of Medicine) To err is human: building a safer health system. Washington, DC: National Academies Press; 1999.

8. The Joint Commission on Accreditation of Healthcare Organizations. 2009 National patient safety goals. Available at: www.jointcommission.org/patientsafety/nationalpatientsafetygoals; 2009. Accessed June 9, 2009.

9. Conroy D. Sterilization. In: Hodge J, Murphy M, editors. Training manual for health care central service technicians. Chicago (IL): Jossey-Bass; 2006. p. 142–77.

10. Conner R. Association of perioperative registered nurses. Standards, recommended practices, and guidelines. 2007 edition. Denver (CO): AORN, Inc; 2007.

11. Denholm B. Clinical issues: malignant hyperthermia; sterilization monitoring; sterilization indicators, multipack needle counts. AORN J 2007;85(2):403–13.

12. Rothrock JC. Infection prevention and control in the perioperative setting. Alexander's care of the patient in surgery. 13th edition. St. Louis (MO): Mosby Elsevier; 2007. p. 75–93.

13. Russell AD, Hugo WB, Ayliffe GA. Principles and practice of disinfection, gaseous sterilization, preservation and sterilization. 3rd edition. Oxford, England: Blackwell Science Ltd; 2001. p. 675–732.

14. Rutala WA. Information on critical issues related to infection control presented during the Eighth Conference on Infectious Diseases. AORN J 2004;80(2):303–10.

15. Seavy R. The need for educated staff in sterile processing—patient safety depends on it. Perioperative Nursing Clinics 2009;4:181–92.

16. American National Standards Institute/Association for the Advancement of Medical Instrumentation. ST58:2005, Chemical sterilization and high-level disinfection in health care facilities. Arlington (VA): Association for the Advancement of Medical Instrumentation; 2006.

17. American National Standards Institute/Association for the Advancement of Medical Instrumentation. ST41:2008, Chemical sterilization and high-level disinfection in health care facilities. Arlington (VA): Association for the Advancement of Medical Instrumentation; 2006.

18. Muscarella LF. Are all sterilization processes alike? AORN J 1998;67(5):966–76.

19. Occupational Health and Safety Administration (OSHA) United States Department of Labor. Regulatory review of the occupational safety and health administration's ozone standard [29 CFR 1910.1000]. Available at: http://www.osha.gov/pls/oshaweb/owadisp.show_document?p_table=STANDARDS&p_id=9992; 2003. Accessed June 9, 2009.

20. Lind N, Ninemeier JD. Low temperature sterilization. In: Lind N, Ninemeier JD, editors. Central service technical manual. 7th edition. Chapter 16. Chicago (IL): International Association of Healthcare Central Service and Material Management; 2008. p. 131–54, 329–42.

21. Rahl R. Understanding oxidative chemistries. Healthcare Purchasing News Online, Available at: www.hpnonline.com; 2006. Accessed June 9, 2009.

22. Murphy L. Ozone—the latest advance in sterilization of medical devices. Can Oper Room Nurs J 2006;24:28–38.

23. Dufresne S, Leblond H, Chaunet M. Relationship between lumen diameter and length sterilized in the 125L ozone sterilizer. Am J Infect Control 2008;36(4):291–7.

Flash Sterilization: A Comprehensive View

Patricia A. Mews, RN, MHA, CNOR

KEYWORDS

• Flash sterilization • Decontamination
• Closed rigid container • Immediate use

IS FLASH STERILIZATION CHANGING? A REVIEW OF CURRENT CONCERNS

Flash sterilization is a topical issue in many operating rooms (ORs), especially those that are challenged with decreasing budgets, reduced reimbursements, the need to improve turnover times, and less ancillary help to assist with non-nursing duties. Simple, basic, general-line instruments are being replaced with complex multipart devices such as flexible endoscopes, microscopic fine instruments, heavy multipart total joint instruments, and robotic instruments. It is much more difficult to ensure that these instruments are clean, functional, and sterile. Another issue of concern is that any breach in the sterilization process can have a direct effect on the patient's recovery and the chance that they may acquire a surgical site infection (SSI). The Never Events compiled by The Center for Medicare and Medicaid Services (CMS) has more stringent rules, and denying payment to health care facilities responsible for SSI and health care–associated infections (HAI) has focused more on sterilization practices by health care facilities.

Patients having surgery anticipate the best possible care during their surgical experience. Perioperative nurses are the patient's advocates to monitor and oversee everything during the surgical intervention that may be adverse to a positive outcome for them. A major responsibility of the perioperative registered nurse is to minimize the patient's risk for SSI by providing surgical items that are free from contaminants at the time of use during their surgical procedure. Flash sterilization may be associated with increased infection risk to patients because of pressure on personnel to eliminate 1 or more steps in the cleaning and sterilization process. Resorting to flash sterilization may ultimately cause the facility more expense and put patients at risk for SSI.[1]

The sterilization process itself is not the concern; it is how the process is performed. John Perkins[2] states that "speed is a militant force against sterilization. It is important to remember that sterilization is an event. It requires the maximum control of all variables so as to affect a minimum margin of doubt in the end result." Flash sterilization implies that sterilization can be achieved instantaneously (in a flash). However, many

Mews Surgical Consulting, 14305 East Cheryl Drive, Scottsdale, AZ 85259, USA
E-mail address: pmews@aol.com

Perioperative Nursing Clinics 5 (2010) 291–326
doi:10.1016/j.cpen.2010.05.004
1556-7931/10/$ – see front matter © 2010 Elsevier Inc. All rights reserved.

periopnursing.theclinics.com

factors can adversely affect the outcome of effective sterilization. Flash sterilization is defined by Association for the Advancement of Medical Instrumentation (AAMI) as the process designed for the steam sterilization of patient-care items for immediate use,[3] and Recommended Practices of The Association of periOperative Registered Nurses (AORN) states that the use of flash sterilization should be kept to a minimum and should be used only in selected clinical situations and in a controlled manner. Flash sterilization should be used only when there is insufficient time to process by the preferred wrapped or container method. Flash sterilization should not be used as a substitute for sufficient instrument inventory. AORN does not recommend flash sterilization because of the lack of quality control and standardized cleaning and processing measures.[4]

Professional organizations define flash sterilization as a process for steam sterilizing instruments and devices for immediate use that have become contaminated (dropped item, compromised wrapper on a one of a kind instrument, chemical indicator [CI] failure), were unanticipated during a procedure, or in an emergency situation. They recommend keeping flash sterilization to a minimum. AAMI states that: "When performed correctly flash sterilization is safe and effective." The emphasis is on correctly and the sterilization process itself is not the concern, but rather how the entire process is performed. The focus should be on what is needed to guarantee that flash sterilization is safe, effective, and will ultimately ensure patient safety. To increase the probability that the item is safe for patient use, it should be required to go through the same conventional sterilization methods that are followed for wrapped and container items.

FLASH STERILIZATION: THE PROCESS IN PERSPECTIVE

Sterilization is the process that kills all forms of microbial life. The concept of what constitutes sterile is measured as the probability of sterility for each item to be sterilized. The probability is known as the sterility assurance level (SAL). For the terminal steam-sterilization process, an SAL of 10^{-6} means that there is less than or equal to 1 chance in 1 million that an item is contaminated or unsterile.[5] The flash sterilization process must achieve the same SAL as terminal sterilization to ensure patient safety. **Table 1** shows AAMI and AORN specific recommendations when considering flash sterilization of instruments or medical devices.

When a surgical team member suggests that an item be flash sterilized for the next patient, they need to consider whether there is another way to sterilize the device. If not, it must be guaranteed that the flash sterilization practices will consistently and successfully follow all the parameters developed by the American National Standards Institute (ANSI)/AAMI, AORN, Association for Practitioners in Infection Control (APIC), and the Centers for Disease Control (CDC) SSI guidelines in order for the surgical patient to receive a positive expected outcome. All conditions must be met before allowing an item to be flash sterilized. Some devices are not suitable for flash sterilization: implants, powered instruments unless specifically approved by manufacturer for flash sterilization processes, and large trays (consignment trays; eg, total joints brought in from outside vendors).

When OR staff members perform flash sterilization practices, their attention may not be focused on the principles of the complete flash sterilization processes. OR staff members must also center their attention on demands from patients and concerns for their safety, surgeons, anesthesia, as well as technical requirements of the surgical procedure. Other concerns include special disposable supplies, maintenance of the sterile field, sponge and instrument counts, documentation, and patient charging.

Table 1
Flash sterilization; recommended practices: flash sterilization may be considered only if all conditions are met

AAMI Recommends	AORN Recommends
• The facility can clean and decontaminate, inspect, and arrange the instruments into the recommended tray or container • The physical design of the area permits delivery of the sterilized devices directly into the procedure room • The facility has developed procedures that are followed and audited to ensure proper handling of devices and safe delivery to the point of use • The item is needed for immediate use following flash sterilization	• The device manufacturer's written instructions on cycle type, exposure times, temperature settings, and drying times are available and followed • Items are disassembled and thoroughly cleaned with detergent and water to remove soil, blood, body fats, and other substances • Lumens are brushed and flushed under water with a cleaning solution, and rinsed thoroughly • Items are placed in a closed sterilization container or tray that is validated for flash sterilization, in a manner that allows steam to contact all instrument surfaces • Measures are taken to prevent contamination during transfer to the sterile field • Flash-sterilized items are to be used immediately and not stored for later use

From ANSI/AAMI ST79:2006 and A2:2009. Comprehensive guide to steam sterilization and sterility assurance in health care facilities. Arlington (VA): Association for the Advancement of Medical Instrumentation. 2009; AORN standards and recommended practices for sterilization in the perioperative practice setting. In: Perioperative standards, recommended practices. Denver (CO): AORN, Inc; 2009. p. 650–3; with permission.

Education is of utmost importance in ensuring that flash sterilization is performed properly, and this can be delegated to ancillary personnel who have been educated and validated in proven competencies.[6]

When flash sterilizing instruments, the primarily concern is on the procedure of cleaning and preparation of instruments for sterilization and the transfer of the sterilized items from the sterilizer to the invasive procedure room using aseptic technique. Increased risks of SSI have been attributed to the process of flash sterilization mainly because the SAL has been compromised by inadequate cleaning of the instrument, or it has become contaminated during transportation or in the presentation to the sterile field. Staff should understand the critical importance of cleaning instruments before subjecting them to any sterilizing process, and should ensure that all steps in the cleaning and sterilizing procedure are consistently followed. The flash sterilization process involves multiple steps and it is important to know whether the device has written instructions from the manufacturer as to whether it can be flash sterilized.

DECONTAMINATION

Most processing and sterilization of instruments and medical devices takes place in the sterile processing department (SPD) outside the OR. Therefore, many OR nurses and surgical technicians are not up to date on the current sterilizing process when they are asked to flash sterilize instruments or devices. The instruments that require a quick turnaround are often sent to SPD for decontamination, cleaning, and assembly and returned to the OR for flash sterilization. When time lines are tight and the OR team waiting for the instruments are demanding a quick turnaround, it is often tempting to shorten the cleaning process. It is critical to follow the complete sterilization process whether performing flash sterilization or terminal sterilization when decontaminating and cleaning all surgical devices to achieve the greatest level of infection prevention. The practice should be standardized and all steps of the cleaning process should be consistent. Research shows that cleaning alone is effective in reducing the number of microorganisms from devices.

Steps to follow are:
- Manufacturers' written instructions for complete reprocessing of devices
- Cleaning and decontamination
- Instrument inspection and assembly
- Sterilizing, monitoring, recording
- Transporting flash-sterilized instruments
- Staff education and competencies
- Quality improvement.

Before any device can be flash sterilized it is important that explicit written instructions from the manufacturer are obtained and followed throughout the reprocessing procedures. The multiple changes in instrument technology and an increase in minimally invasive procedures using more complex, fine, and delicate instruments impose a greater challenge to render devices sterile to ensure patient safety and prevent the risk of SSI.

AORN's recommended practices for cleaning and care of surgical instruments and powered equipment involves 22 steps (**Table 2**). These steps are necessary because they are the most critical in breaking the chain of infection and disease. Effective cleaning is a prerequisite to effective sterilization and disinfection. Ineffective decontamination and cleaning can comprise sterilization and have been associated with adverse patient outcomes.[7]

Some facilities may take an abbreviated approach to flash sterilizing surgical instruments, but devices to be flashed sterilized should be subjected to the same cleaning and decontamination processes as described in **Table 2**. If this approach to flash sterilization does not include the proper practice of each step of the sterilization processes recommended by AORN, including proper decontamination, cleaning, and transportation of the sterilized items to the point of use, patients may be at risk for an SSI. Perioperative nurses should understand the critical importance of cleaning instruments before subjecting them to any sterilizing process and ensure that all the steps in the cleaning and sterilizing procedure are consistently followed. The most essential step of the flash sterilization process is the cleaning and decontamination of the items. This step reduces bioburden and removes all visible and invisible soil and blood from items before they are handled. It is critical because soil must be removed before instruments are ready for assembly and sterilization. Soil/bioburden can interfere with, or even prevent, the achievement of sterilization. The Occupational Safety and Health Administration[8] (OSHA) defines decontamination as the use of physical or chemical means to remove, inactivate, or destroy blood-borne pathogens on a surface or item to the point at which they are no longer capable of transmitting infectious particles, and the surface or item is rendered safe for handling, use, or disposal.

Decontamination is defined by AORN[9] as any physical or chemical process that removes or reduces the number of microorganisms or infectious agents and renders reusable medical products or equipment safe for handling or disposal; the process by which contaminants are removed, by hand cleaning or mechanical means, using

Table 2
Recommended practices for cleaning and care of surgical instruments and powered equipment

1. The manufacturer's written, validated instructions for handling and reprocessing should be obtained and evaluated to determine the ability to adequately clean and reprocess the equipment within the health care facility before purchasing surgical instruments and powered equipment
2. New, repaired, and refurbished instruments should be examined, cleaned, and sterilized according to manufacturers' written instructions before use in health care organization
3. Borrowed or consigned (ie, loaner) instruments should be examined, cleaned, and sterilized by the receiving health care organization before use, according to manufacturers' written instructions
4. Instruments should be kept free from gross soil during surgical procedures
5. Cleaning and decontamination should occur as soon as possible after instruments and equipment are used
6. Contaminated instruments must be contained during transport and should be transported in a timely manner to a location designed for decontamination
7. Instruments should be decontaminated in an area separate from locations where clean activities are performed
8. The type of water available for cleaning should be consistent with the manufacturer's written instructions and the intended use of the equipment and cleaning agent
9. Surgical instrument, medical device, and equipment manufacturers' validated instructions should be followed regarding the types of cleaning agents (eg, enzyme preparations, detergents) to be used for decontamination
10. All surgical instrument and medical device or equipment manufacturers' validated instructions should be followed regarding the types of cleaning methods (eg, manual, automated) to be used for decontamination
11. Surgical instruments should be inspected for cleanliness and proper working order after decontamination
12. Cleaned surgical instruments should be organized for packaging in a manner to allow the sterilant to contact all exposed surfaces
13. Powered surgical instruments and all attachments should be decontaminated, lubricated, assembled, sterilized, and tested before use according to the manufacturer's written instructions
14. Special precautions should be taken for reprocessing ophthalmic surgical instruments
15. Insulated electrosurgery instruments should be decontaminated after use according to manufacturers' validated, written instructions, and inspected for damage
16. Special precautions should be taken when cleaning robotic instruments
17. Special precautions should be taken to minimize the risk of transmission of prion diseases
18. Personnel handling contaminated instruments and equipment must wear appropriate personal protective equipment and should be vaccinated against the hepatitis B virus
19. Personnel should receive initial education and competency validation on procedures, chemicals used, and personal protection, and should receive additional training when new equipment, instruments, supplies, or procedures are introduced
20. Documentation should be completed to enable the identification of trends and to demonstrate compliance with regulatory and accrediting agency requirements
21. Policies and procedures regarding the care and cleaning of surgical instruments and powered equipment should be developed using the validated instructions provided by the medical device manufacturers, reviewed at regular intervals, revised as necessary, and be readily available in the practice setting
22. The health care organization's quality management program should evaluate the care of instruments to improve patient safety

From Recommended practices for cleaning and care of surgical instruments and power equipment. In: Perioperative standards, recommended practices. Denver (CO): AORN, Inc; 2009. p. 611–35; with permission.

specific solutions capable of rendering blood and debris harmless and removing them from the surface of an object or instrument.

AAMI's guidelines state that the type of decontamination required for a particular contaminated device depends on the biohazard that the device presents. The cleaning or microbicidal process appropriate for a particular device depends on the following:

- The device manufacturer's written instructions
- The necessary level of microbial kill; for example, a higher assurance of lethality is needed for items that have been in contact with body tissues, blood, or body fluids than for items that have only been in contact with unbroken skin
- The design of the device; for example, items that have been contaminated with blood or body fluids and that have sharp points or edges capable of puncturing or abrading the skin should be subjected to a decontamination process that includes disinfection or sterilization
- Other characteristics of the device; for example, whether the materials from which the device is fabricated can tolerate high temperatures or whether the device is fully immersible.

Health care personnel, including representatives of Sterile Processing and Infection Control, should make a concerted effort to purchase only those devices that can be decontaminated appropriately by a method available in the health care facility. Device manufacturers have the responsibility to provide complete and comprehensive written instructions for the decontamination of their products, as well as a summary and interpretation of test results verifying that their products can be safely and effectively decontaminated.[10]

The decontamination area should be separate from areas in which the procedures are performed and surgical instruments sterilized. Proper cleaning requires more than wiping and soaking of instruments on the sterile field or a quick wash or rinse in the scrub sink. Soiled instruments should never be cleaned with brushes intended for surgical hand antisepsis, and cleaning soiled instruments in a scrub or hand sink can contaminate the sink and faucet. Physical separation of clean activities from decontamination and cleaning of instruments avoids the possibility of cross-contamination. Hand washing is the single most important action for preventing HAI in patients and staff members, therefore hand washing and instrument cleaning should never be permitted in the same sink.[11]

The decontamination area should have

- A door that remains closed and contains the equipment
- Sinks to manually clean instruments
- Hand-washing facilities, and an eye-wash station
- Automated equipment consistent with the types of instruments to be decontaminated
- A compressed air supply.[9]

Patient and staff safety are of concern and depend on the proper reprocessing of instruments and staff education and protection. Organizations, agencies, and facilities are concerned about staff safety during the decontamination and cleaning process, therefore policies and procedures should be followed precisely. Staff involved in the cleaning and decontamination process of contaminated devices should use personal protective equipment (PPE) and should be vaccinated against the hepatitis B virus.[12]

PPE helps to protect staff from exposure to blood-borne pathogens and other potentially infectious materials. Splashes, splatters, and skin contact can be anticipated when handling contaminated instruments. Appropriate PPE for these types of exposures include, but are not limited to, a fluid-resistant gown, disposable head cover to contain all hair, heavy-duty gloves, and face protection including eye protection such as goggles or a full face shield. Having PPE readily available at the point of use encourages staff to wear it regardless of the number of instruments to be cleaned. Transport soiled instruments to the decontamination area in a manner that prevents contamination of the personnel and environment. On arrival in the decontamination area, contaminated items should be removed from their transport containers, sorted, disassembled, and prepared for cleaning. All instruments should be thoroughly cleaned and rinsed following the device manufacturers' written instructions.

CLEANING OF DEVICES

Cleaning is defined by AAMI as the removal of contamination from an item to the extent necessary for further processing or for the intended use. AAMI notes that: "...cleaning consists of the removal, usually with detergent and water, of adherent soil (eg, blood, protein, and other debris) from the surfaces, crevices, serrations, joints and lumens of instruments, devices and equipment by a manual or mechanical process that prepares the items for safe handling and or further decontamination." Cleaning removes microbial contamination and organic and inorganic material, which, if not removed, can interfere with sterilization or disinfection. Cleaning should begin as soon as possible after an item is used. Precleaning and sorting begins in the OR at the sterile field with the scrub person keeping instruments free from gross soil during the surgical procedure by wiping with a sponge moistened with sterile water. Blood, tissue, or mucus that is allowed to dry on surgical instruments is difficult to remove and will lengthen the time necessary to clean the instrument effectively. It may also cause pitting, rusting, or corrosion. Saline should not be used for removing debris because it can cause deterioration of instrument surfaces. Irrigate instrument lumens with sterile water throughout the procedure to keep patent. Cleaning steps should be standardized and consistent. Instruments should be categorized according to the appropriate cleaning process to assist personnel in selecting cleaning methods and to reduce the risk of instrument damage and staff injury. Disassembly, physical cleaning, and decontamination of the device are the initial and most critical steps in breaking the chain of disease transmission. Pay particular attention to difficult-to-clean areas that include box locks, serrations, hinges, crevices, lumens, and devices such as flexible reamers and biopsy forceps where debris can easily be trapped and go unnoticed.

The goal is to remove soil and reduce the bioburden on all devices by thorough cleaning and copious rinsing according to the manufacturer's instructions. Debris, blood, mucous, and tissue will interfere with the sterilization process, and sterilization will not compensate for poor or inadequate cleaning. Instruments that go through sterilization and have even the smallest amounts of debris remaining on them cannot be considered sterile. Proper mechanical or hand decontamination and cleaning, depending on the device, is essential in removing bioburden and preparing devices for sterilization. Verification and documentation of the cleaning process are essential, and manufacturers should provide test procedures that can be easily replicated and that can help users recognize whether cleaning was effective for all device areas. Such tests are important for devices with components that cannot be readily inspected for cleanliness (eg, spring hinges, lumens, porous materials, crevices). Failures in instrument cleaning have resulted in transmission of infectious agents.[13]

Most sterilization failures result from inadequate cleaning of the instruments before sterilization.

EYE INSTRUMENT CONCERNS: TOXIC ANTERIOR SEGMENT SYNDROME

The cleaning of intraocular surgical instruments has caused concern because of the increasingly reported complication of cataract surgery as a result of toxic anterior segment syndrome (TASS). TASS is a sterile postoperative inflammatory reaction in the anterior chamber of the eye that can cause damage to intraocular tissues and lead to permanent corneal endothelial and iris damage, an irregular dilated pupil, and increased intraocular pressure resulting in secondary glaucoma.[14] Cataract surgery is one of the most common surgical procedures performed in the United States for patients 65 years of age and older. Although adverse events after cataract surgery are rare, they can include infectious and noninfectious complications. The causes of TASS have involved several factors, one of which is the processing/care and handling of intraocular surgical instruments. Most cases of TASS seem to result from inadequate instrument cleaning and sterilization.[15]

Because of the quick turnaround time that cataract surgeries demand and the lack of adequate instrumentation, steps in the sterilization process are skipped. Intraocular surgical instruments are the most common instruments that are flashed sterilized and, because of the hurriedness of the environment, many steps in the cleaning and sterilization process are overlooked. Flash sterilization has been attributed to TASS because of inadequate cleaning and processing of the instruments used during cataract surgery. As a consequence of inadequate or inappropriate instrument cleaning, irritants on the surfaces of intraocular surgical instruments have accumulated (denatured ophthalmic viscosurgical devices [OVDs]).[16] Therefore, special consideration in the cleaning of intraocular instruments should be considered. Preventing TASS requires appropriate management of intraocular surgical instruments and must be repeated with each phase of decontamination, cleaning, and sterilization of intraocular surgical instruments wherever cataract surgery is performed. **Table 3** lists recommendations for cleaning and sterilizing intraocular surgical instruments developed by the American Society of Cataract and Refractive Surgery (ASCRS) TASS Task Force. Perioperative managers must understand that cleaning is the most critical step in any reprocessing procedure and ensure that staff members are adequately trained to effectively and consistently perform this task. Most importantly, manufacturer's written instructions for cleaning each instrument should be reviewed and followed. Adequate time should be provided to allow completion of all steps of cleaning and sterilization. Staff training, competency validation, and periodic performance review should be implemented for each health care facility. They should also understand that, in emergencies when flash sterilization is used in addition to the multistep cleaning process, they must ensure that the correct cycle is selected (eg, 3 minutes at 132°C in a gravity-displacement sterilizer for instruments without lumens or porous materials and 10 minutes for instruments with lumens and porous material). Records should be maintained of all cleaning methods; detergent solutions used, and lot numbers of cleaning solutions. These records can be used to facilitate investigation of any suspected or confirmed cases of TASS. An adequate inventory of instruments should be provided to allow for thorough instrument cleaning and sterilization. These requirements facilitate compliance with proper decontamination and sterilization processes and avoid flash sterilization.[9]

ASSEMBLY AND INSPECTION

Before assembly of trays, and after cleaning, inspect instruments that may require repairs or additional cleaning. Inspecting devices for function and under lighted magnification also identifies additional concerns that may need further attention. Insulated instruments should be tested for their intactness to prevent patient burns during use. While assembling instruments in a tray, organize them in a manner that will allow the sterilant to contact all exposed surfaces. Positioning the items in the tray or container in a manner that allows steam to contact all instrument surfaces is an important part of the process. Air removal, steam penetration, and drainage of condensate are all affected by proper positioning. Drainage of condensate is important because flash sterilization does not provide for drying of items. Positioning of items to reduce puddling of moisture is critical. All hinged instruments should be opened, multiple-part devices should be disassembled, and items with lumens should be flushed with distilled water immediately before sterilization only if specified by the manufacturer. Delicate and sharp instruments should be protected using tip protectors or positioned within a container that stabilizes the instruments with pegs, racks, or stringers. Use only containment devices validated for flash sterilization according to the manufacturer's specific instructions to organize or position instruments within trays.

RIGID FLASH-STERILIZATION CONTAINERS

Not all containers are approved or tested for flash sterilization. Only containers specifically designed for flash sterilization cycles, and cleared by the Food and Drug Administration (FDA), should be used. Closed rigid containers designated for flash sterilization provide the following:

- Reduced risk of contamination during transport to the point of use
- Ease of presentation to the sterile field
- Protection of sterilized items during transport
- The ability to be opened, used immediately, and not stored for later use
- The ability to be differentiated from other types of containers used for terminal sterilization
- The ability to be used, cleaned, and maintained according to the manufacturer's written instructions.[4]

Obtain documentation and instructions for use from the container manufacturer for flash sterilization of that specific container device, to include the parameters required to achieve sterilization as well as any load or chamber capacity limits such as weight, contents, and configuration. Manufacturers are responsible for providing users with documentation of testing and validation studies performed and a comprehensive instruction manual. The facility should be able to verify the manufacturer's results. Manufacturers should provide documentation for approved devices (power equipment, items with lumens, maximum weight of instruments) that may be placed inside the container for flash sterilization. Follow ANSI/AAMI ST79:2006-A2.2009 guidelines for the evaluation and testing of sealed flash containers in your facility. Regardless of whether the items are wrapped or containerized, they are intended for immediate use and cannot be stored for later use. Flashed closed, rigid containers and single-wrapped/packaged trays often look similar to containers intended for terminal sterilization, but they are not interchangeable. Special precautions should be taken to ensure that these closed, rigid containers and single-wrapped/packaged trays are distinguished from conventional terminal sterilization containers and trays.

Table 3
American Society of Cataract and Refractive Surgery (ASCRS) TASS Task Force recommended practices for cleaning and sterilizing intraocular surgical instruments

1. Adequate time for thorough cleaning and sterilization of instrumentation should be established
   Flash sterilization is designed to manage unanticipated, urgent needs for instruments. Flash sterilization should not be used to save time or as a substitute for sufficient instrument inventory

2. For each piece of equipment, the manufacturer's direction for use (DFU) pertaining to cleaning and sterilization should be followed

3. OVD solution, which can dry and harden within minutes, should not be allowed to dry on the instruments

4. Whether or not they are used, instruments opened for a procedure should be transported from the OR in a closed container to the decontamination area, where cleaning should be completed immediately

5. Disposable cannulas and tubing should be used whenever possible, and they should be discarded after each use

6. Devices labeled for single use only should not be reused; single-use devices do not include instructions for reuse or reprocessing. The US Food and Drug Administration (FDA) actively regulates third-party and hospital reprocessors of single-use devices

7. To avoid contamination with bioburden and cleaning chemicals, intraocular instruments should be cleaned separately from nonophthalmologic surgical instruments

8. The importance of enzymatic detergents for the cleaning of soiled intraocular instruments has not been established. Inappropriate use and incomplete rinsing of enzymatic detergents have been associated with outbreaks of TASS

9. If an ultrasonic cleaner is used, follow ultrasonic and instrument manufacturer's DFU during the entire process

10. Manual cleaning processes: cleaning tools should be designed for cleaning medical instruments
    Disposable cleaning apparatus should be discarded after each use and reusable items should be cleaned and high-level disinfected or sterilized
    Cleaning solutions should be discarded after each use
    When flushing is used as part of the cleaning, the effluent should be discarded and not reused

11. Unless otherwise specified by the manufacturer's DFU, sterile distilled, or sterile deionized, water should be used for the final rinse of instruments
    Rinsing should provide a flow of water through or over instruments, with effluent discarded as it is used; use only debris-free water for rinsing
    Agitation in a basin of water should not be used as a final rinse

12. Instruments with lumens should be dried with forced or compressed air. Compressed air should be filtered and free from oil and water. Instruments with lumens should be fully dried

13. Specific instruments: phacoemulsifier handpiece, irrigator/aspirator, irrigator/aspirator tips, and inserters:

Flush phacoemulsifier handpiece with balanced saline solution before removing from the operative field

Wipe each instrument with a lint-free cloth and place immediately in a bath of sterile water. Remove from the operative field and remove from sites that maintain instruments needed for completion of the surgical procedure, in strict accordance with the manufacturer's DFU for each piece of equipment. To avoid introduction of water, or reintroduction of gross soil, to the operative field, the sterile water bath should be clearly separated from the operative field

Clean and flush each item in accordance with the manufacturer's DFU and verify removal of all debris inclusive of OVD

Inspect irrigator/aspirator tips, preferably under magnification, before sterilization

14. If reusable woven materials are used for draping the sterile field, to absorb condensate in steam sterilized instrument trays or to wipe instruments, they should be laundered and rinsed thoroughly between each use to eliminate surgical compounds, debris, and cleaning agents

Laundry procedures should be reviewed and monitored to ensure delivery of residue-free, reused woven materials; otherwise disposable, chemical, and lint-free materials should be used

All woven materials used in intraocular surgery or instrument management should be lint free

15. Cleanliness and integrity of instruments should be verified

Instruments should be visually inspected for debris and damage, preferably under magnification, immediately after cleaning and before packaging for sterilization to ensure removal of visible debris

Additional or repeated cleaning and rinsing steps may be required on a case-by-case basis to ensure removal of all debris and OVD

Surgeons should examine instruments under the microscope before each use and reject any instrument that shows signs of residual debris or defects

16. The method for sterilizing intraocular surgical instruments should be in accordance with the DFU of the instruments and with the DFU of the sterilizer manufacturer

Steam sterilization should be completed in accordance with published guidelines

Glutaraldehyde is not recommended for sterilizing intraocular instruments because of the toxicity of glutaraldehyde residues resulting from inadequate rinsing or contamination during poststerilization handling

Other low-temperature methods of sterilization should not be used unless the ophthalmic instrument manufacturer and the sterilizer manufacturer have validated the method for the specific instruments with respect to efficacy of sterilization, potential ocular toxicity (eg, from oxidation of metals), and instrument functionality

Verification of sterilizer function should be completed at least weekly (preferably daily), in accordance with the sterilizer manufacturer's instructions for use and with published guidelines, and documented in the facility log

Measures should be taken to ensure that preventive maintenance, cleaning, and inspection of sterilizers are performed on a scheduled basis, according to the sterilizer manufacturer's written instructions. All preventive maintenance should be documented

Maintenance of boilers, of the water filtration systems, and of the quality of water supplying the steam-sterilizing system should be verified at least yearly

(continued on next page)

Table 3
(continued)

17. Administrative controls, such as policies and procedures regarding cleaning and sterilizing intraocular surgical instruments, should be implemented
    Sufficient instrument sets and equipment should be available to allow adequate time for cleaning and sterilization between procedures
    Personnel should be educated about TASS and its causes and should receive initial education, training, and validation of competency in the cleaning, inspection, preparation, packaging, sterilization, storage, and distribution of all intraocular surgical instruments. Education, training and validation of competency should be updated at least annually and before introduction of any new devices or procedures
    Records of instrument use, of medication use, and of sterilization should be maintained in accordance with facility policy. Complete and detailed records will aid in the investigation of any occurrence of TASS
    AORN

Statement from the Academy and ASCRS regarding the Joint Commission's clarification of its position on sterilization practices. Recently, there has been concern and confusion about the interpretation of standards and survey process regarding sterilization in ophthalmic facilities. Over the past year, the American Academy of Ophthalmology (Academy) and the American Society of Cataract and Refractive Surgery (ASCRS), along with the Outpatient Ophthalmic Surgical Society, have discussed the concerns of ophthalmic surgery centers with the Joint Commission. The new position statement released by the Joint Commission on June 15, 2009, www.jointcommission.org, further discusses the standards regarding steam sterilization.

From TASS Special report: Recommended practices for cleaning and sterilizing intraocular surgical instruments. American Society of Cataract and Refractive Surgery, American Society of Ophthalmic Registered Nurses, ASCRS TASS Task Force; use in conjunction with AAMI (Association for the Advancement of Medical Instrumentation) the American Society of Ophthalmic Registered Nurses (ASORN), and the Association of periOperative Registered Nurses (AORN)[33]; prepared February 16, 2007, by the American Society of Cataract and Refractive Surgery Ad Hoc Task Force on Cleaning and Sterilization of Intraocular Instruments. Guidance provided by the Association of periOperative Registered Nurses, the Association for Professionals in Infection Control and Epidemiology, the Society for Healthcare Epidemiology of America, the Centers for Disease Control and Prevention, and the US Food and Drug Administration; with permission.

TRANSPORTING STERILE ITEMS
Open Tray

In an emergent situation when a closed container is unavailable and an open tray is used, it is not the efficacy of the flash sterilization that is in question but the ability to safely deliver the unwrapped sterilized items to the sterile field without contamination. Transferring the sterilized item to the sterile field without contamination is difficult and should be based on the assumption that condensate will be present within the tray, so care should be taken to avoid contamination of the sterilized items. The tray, and the items within it, will also be hot, so care should be taken to avoid thermal injury. The scrubbed individual transporting the sterile device must be alert to all sources of potential contamination. If the sterilizer is within a substerile room connected to an OR, the circulating nurse directs (while opening doors) the scrub person donned in sterile attire to the substerile room. Using folded sterile towels like potholders to protect from burns, the scrub person retrieves the sterilized tray, and returns to the room, placing it on a sterile field. The tray should never be placed on a nonsterile surface. Meticulous conscientiousness is required from the circulator and scrub person to avoid any contamination to the scrub's sterile attire or the sterilized tray during the transportation. Patient safety should be of utmost importance and, because the instruments are hot, they should not be used until they are cooled. It is particularly important that the flash sterilization method of steam-sterilization processing be performed in a clean environment and that devices processed by this method be transferred and handled as little as possible, because the items are not protected by packaging before or after the sterilization process.[17] This practice should be audited and monitored to provide for aseptic handling and personnel safety during transport of the sterilized items.

Single-wrapped Trays

Some prevacuum and pulsing gravity-displacement steam sterilizers have a cycle that is designed to permit prevacuum flash sterilization using a single, nonwoven or textile wrapper. The parameters for this sterilization cycle are established or preset by the sterilizer manufacturer and vary depending on the design of the sterilizer. This cycle is designed for flash sterilization of all-metal, nonporous items only (except for the wrapper), arranged on a perforated or mesh-bottom instrument tray. Items with lumens, or complex medical devices, cannot be processed in this cycle because air removal and steam contact within them may not be achieved; this cycle has fewer prevacuum pulses than a regular prevacuum cycle. On some sterilizers, this cycle is called the express cycle. It operates in the same way as the prevacuum cycle, in that it uses mechanical air removal; however, there are only 2 injections of steam and chamber evacuations before the exposure temperature is reached. Following the exposure time, steam is exhausted and a brief dry time is used. The preset exposure time on sterilizers with express cycles is 4 minutes at 132°C, followed by a 3 minute dry time. The total cycle time is about 12 minutes. The single wrapper protects the sterilized items from environmental contamination that may be encountered en route from the sterilizer to the point of use. These single-wrapped flash-sterilized trays must be used immediately. However, precautions must be taken to differentiate these single-wrapped flash-sterilized trays from other wrapped trays that have been terminally processed.[18]

Procedures for transferring the items from the sterilizer to the point of use should be based on the assumption that condensate will be present within the container and that the items within the wrapper will be hot. Although the outer wrapper may seem to be dry, there will be condensation within the tray. Moisture can strike through the wrapper or other packaging, so care should be taken to avoid contamination by contact with nonsterile surfaces. Personnel should wear sterile gloves and may use sterile towels as potholders when removing items from the sterilizer. The wrapped/packaged tray should never be placed on a nonsterile surface. A sterile, impervious drape, placed on a surface separate from the sterile field, should be used so that the wrapped/packaged tray can be placed there and then opened by the circulator. The sterile items may then be removed from the tray by the scrub person and taken to the sterile field. However, at the end of the cycle the wrapper or other packaging could be wet on the bottom, depending on the amount of condensation created by the types and number of instruments within the tray. The wrapper or other packaging may seem dry when the sterilizer is opened, but handling of the wrapped/packaged item can cause the wrapper or other packaging to become wet in places.[17]

Sealed Rigid Containers

Flash sterilization should be achieved using a rigid closed container specifically designed and intended for flash sterilization cycles and cleared by the FDA. Rigid flash-sterilization containers accomplish the following:

- Reduced risk of contamination during transport to the point of use
- Ease of presentation to the sterile field
- Protection of sterilized items during transport.

Flash-sterilization containers should be used, cleaned, and maintained according to the manufacturer's written instructions. They should be opened, used immediately, and not stored for later use. These containers should be differentiated from other types of sterilization containers.[4] There are several different types of rigid closed containers especially designed for flash sterilization. AAMI recommends that flash-sterilization containers be tested in each facility's sterilizer to verify that sterilization can be achieved when used in that particular sterilizer. It is important that the manufacturer of the containers provide written, scientific documentation that its containers are suitable for the flash sterilization process. When the flash sterilization cycle is complete, and before the sterilized device is removed from the sterilizer, the operator needs to ensure that parameters of time and temperature required for sterilization have been met by reviewing and initialing the sterilizer printout. Once verified, the closed container (which may need to be closed after the cycle, depending on the type) protects the sterilized device during transport to the operative/invasive procedure room. Procedures for transferring the items from the sterilizer to the point of use should be based on the assumption that condensate will be present within the container and that it is hot (as is typical of flash sterilization). Personnel may wear sterile gloves or use sterile towels as potholders when removing items from the sterilizer. The containerized items should never be placed on a nonsterile surface.[19] A sterile, impervious drape, placed on a surface separate from the sterile field (back table), should be used and then opened by the circulator. The sterile items may be removed from the container by the scrub person and taken to the sterile field. This type of flash cycle includes a brief drying time. However, at the end of the cycle the interior of the containment device could be wet on the bottom, depending on the amount of condensation created by the types and number of instruments being sterilized.[17]

Policy and procedures should be developed in consultation with perioperative management and the infection control professional, with the objective of ensuring the best practice possible for aseptic transfer within the physical constraints of the facility.

Many ORs are designed with flash sterilizers opening into a common hallway through which clean and dirty case carts, patient stretchers, and all staff members travel. This OR design poses a challenge, especially when transporting sterile devices to the OR/procedure room. It is critical that any devices that are flash sterilized in this kind of environment must be in a closed rigid container designed for flash sterilization to avoid contamination from the busy surroundings within the hallway. Sterilizers used for flash sterilization should be located within the restricted areas of the operative/invasive areas where procedures are performed, such as substerile rooms or the sterile supply core of the OR. It is most important to select the correct cycle parameters for the devices to be flash sterilized. These exposure times and temperature settings should be selected according to the device, container, and the sterilizer manufacturers' written instructions. The flash sterilization cycle can be affected by the sterilizer model, design, age, steam source, method of air removal, and sterilizer maintenance. Exposure times may vary and staff should obtain documentation from the manufacturer that includes flash sterilization validation for wrapped trays, rigid containers along with instructions on how to use, and the parameters required to achieve sterilization, as well as any load or chamber capacity limits such as weight, contents configuration, and other restrictions. **Table 4** indicates recommended minimum cycle times for flash sterilization.

In modern ORs there are several types of steam sterilizers used for flash sterilization. Historically, gravity-displacement sterilizers were the only types that flash-sterilized instruments. Steam sterilizers vary in design and performance characteristics. Some examples are gravity-displacement cycles, dynamic air removal (prevacuum), steam-flush pressure-pulse cycles, flash cycles, and express cycles (ie, abbreviated steam-sterilization cycles used for flash sterilization). In addition, some sterilizers may be designed to permit only one type of cycle. For example, some sterilizers are identified as gravity-displacement sterilizers because they only permit that type of cycle. With new technology and state-of-the-art equipment, 1 sterilizer can typically perform different cycles for flash sterilization. Knowledge of sterilization operating instructions is essential in identifying and understanding the basics of sterilization. Understanding the composition and function of steam sterilizers helps to comprehend why the process is so critical, and takes more than 3 or 10 minutes from start to finish of a cycle. All steam sterilizers have 3 phases: the conditioning, exposure, and exhaust phase.

The gravity-displacement cycle is the most commonly used cycle for flash sterilization.

Conditioning Phase:
- Steam comes from the source and enters the sterilizer jacket (the space between the sterilizer chamber wall and the outer shell)
- Steam enters the sterilizing chamber from the jacket and forms a layer above the air
- Steam is continually admitted and the air is pushed out through the chamber drain. It is important that all of the air be removed, because it can prevent steam from contacting the surfaces that are to be sterilized
- As air is pushed out, the load is heated and the chamber temperature is sensed by the temperature probe in the chamber drain line
- When all of the air is pushed out, the trap closes
- Pressure increases inside the chamber, allowing the chamber to achieve sterilizing temperature
- Once the preselected sterilizing temperature is reached, the exposure phase begins.

Table 4
Examples of typical flash steam-sterilization parameters

Type of Sterilizer	Load Configuration	Time (min)	Exposure Temperature (°C)	Drying Times (min)
Gravity displacement	Metal or nonporous items only (ie, no lumens)	3	132–135	0–1
	Metal items with lumens and porous items (eg, rubber, plastic) sterilized together. Complex devices (eg, powered instruments requiring extended exposure times). Manufacturer instructions should be consulted	10	132–135	0–1
Dynamic air removal (prevacuum)	Metal or nonporous items only (ie, no lumens)	3	132–135	N/A
	Metal items with lumens and porous items sterilized together	4	132	N/A
		3	135	N/A

The sterilizer manufacturer's instructions for use of express cycles should be followed. One sterilizer manufacturer provides an express flash cycle that permits flash sterilization with a single-ply wrapper to help contain the device to the point of use. This cycle is not recommended for devices with lumens. Express cycles should only be used if the sterilizer is designed with this feature.

Steam-flush pressure pulse: see manufacturers' written instructions for time and temperature.

This table does not include specific instructions for rigid flash-sterilization containers. The container manufacturer's instructions should be followed.

From Association for the Advancement of Medical Instrumentation. ANSI/AAMI ST79:2006:A2:2009. Comprehensive guide to steam sterilization and sterility assurance in health care facilities. Arlington (VA); Association for the Advancement of Medical Instrumentation; 2006: A2:2009:8.6.2.1,2,3.4,5. p. 70–1. AORN standards and recommended practices for sterilization in the perioperative practice setting. In: Perioperative standards and recommended practices. Denver (CO): AORN, Inc; 2009. p. 652; with permission.

Exposure Phase:

This phase lasts for the amount of time that has been set for a particular item to be sterilized.

Unwrapped, nonporous, all-metal surgical instruments

    3 minutes at 132–135°C

Unwrapped mixed porous and nonporous items: rubber, plastic, lumen, multiparts

    10 minutes at 132–135°C

At the completion of the exposure phase, the exhaust phase begins.

Exhaust Phase:

- Steam is removed from the chamber
- Sterilizer chamber is brought back to atmospheric pressure
- Atmospheric pressure and a small vacuum may be pulled to remove excess steam from the chamber
- Air is reintroduced through a filter that removes contaminants
- End-of-cycle signal sounds, signaling that the chamber door can be opened.

DYNAMIC AIR-REMOVAL (PREVACUUM) CYCLE

Flash sterilization can also be accomplished in sterilizers with prevacuum cycles, also known as prevac sterilizers. In a prevacuum cycle, air is mechanically pulled from the chamber during the conditioning phase and steam is actively pulled out during the exhaust phase at the end of the sterilizing cycle. Mechanical air removal is accomplished using a vacuum pump or an ejector system, which is more efficient than the gravity-displacement method. During this process, there are several injections of steam. Each injection is followed by a chamber evacuation to remove steam and air. Once the appropriate injections and evacuations are complete and the appropriate exposure temperature is reached, the steam pressure is held for the appropriate sterilizing time and then exhausted. A dry time may be used if desired.

Routine exposure parameters for prevacuum cycles are as follows:

Nonporous cycle for surface sterilization; all-metal surgical instruments

    3 minutes at 132–135°C

Porous cycle; rubber, plastic, lumen or multiparts, combined metal instruments, and porous items

    4 minutes at 132–135°C. This cycle can be shortened because of the more efficient air removal, steam penetration, and contact of steam with the items to be sterilized

Longer exposure times may be required by the manufacturers of some complex medical devices.[18]

STEAM-STERILIZATION MEASURES OF STERILITY ASSURANCE

AAMI recommends routine monitoring of steam sterilizers at least weekly, preferably daily at the beginning of each day the steam sterilizer is used, to ascertain whether the sterilizer is functioning properly. The foundation of a successful sterilization process monitoring program is the process by which a load is monitored and released based on the results of a biologic indicator (BI) in a process challenge device (PCD).

PROCESS MONITORING PCDS

Every load that is sterilized should be physically monitored to verify cycle parameters. A class 1 CI should be placed externally on every item and an internal CI for class 3, 4, or 5 should be placed inside the item. PCDs are used to test the different functions of sterilizers to validate the accurate mechanism of any steam sterilizer and assess whether items have been exposed to sufficient conditions for sterilization. A PCD is used to assess the effective performance of a sterilization process by providing a challenge to the process that is equal to or greater than the challenge posed by the most difficult item routinely processed. Each sterilizer cycle must be monitored. Commercial PCDs intended for use in health care facilities should be approved by the FDA. Manufacturers of PCDs should provide written instructions for the use, storage, handling, and testing of their products. When selecting a commercial PCD, health care personnel should ask the manufacturer the following questions:

- Is the PCD appropriate for the specific steam-sterilization cycle being used?
- Has the performance of the PCD been shown to be equivalent to the performance of the user-assembled challenge test pack?
- What types of BIs or CIs are used in the PCD?
- Can this PCD be used for routine sterilizer efficacy monitoring and sterilizer qualification testing, or is it only suitable for use in routine load release?
- If the monitor in the PCD indicates a questionable sterilization cycle, what procedure should be followed to investigate the potential sterilization process failure?
- Does the PCD have a specific shelf life? What are the specific storage requirements for the PCD?[20]

EQUIPMENT CONTROL: PHYSICAL MONITORING

Equipment control involves sterilizer monitoring before the first load of the day and continues with each cycle during the day to ascertain that the sterilizer is functioning at the programmed settings of time, temperature, pressure, and sterilant exposure. Physical monitors record cycle parameters such as time and temperature for each cycle. The physical monitoring devices include computerized digital printouts, grafts, and gauges and they can indicate immediate sterilization failure. Physical monitoring provides real-time assessment of the sterilization cycle conditions and provides permanent records by means of chart recordings or printouts. Physical monitoring will not detect loading and packaging problems that can interfere with steam sterilization because these monitors only measure the chamber temperature and not the temperature inside each package. Some sterilizers provide printouts that should be checked to verify that the cycle identification number has been recorded and that the pen or printer is functioning properly. For sterilizers with recording charts, check that at the beginning of the cycle the chart is marked with the correct date and sterilizer number. At the end of the cycle and before items are removed from the sterilizer, examine and interpret the printout or chart to confirm that all cycle parameters were met and initial it to permit later identification of the operator. Cycle information and monitoring results must be documented to allow the opportunity to track the item to the individual patient on whom it was used.

ROUTINE MONITORING WITH BOWIE-DICK TEST (EQUIPMENT CONTROL)

If the sterilizer performs gravity-displacement and dynamic air-removal (prevacuum) cycles then both cycles should be tested daily. Routine testing on all sterilizers should be conducted each day the sterilizers are used and at the same time every day before the first process load to assess whether the sterilizer is functioning properly. **Table 5** lists step-by-step guidelines for routine sterilizer testing and acceptance criteria. All dynamic air-removal (prevacuum) sterilizers, whether used for flash sterilization or not, should be tested daily beginning with a Bowie-Dick (B-D) test pack that contains a class 2 CI. The test should be run in accordance with the test manufacturer's instructions before routine BI testing. It provides evidence that the air vacuum pump in dynamic air-removal (prevacuum) sterilizers is removing air efficiently before the start of daily routine sterilization. If the sterilizer has an inadequate vacuum, an air leak, or poor steam quality, air pockets form inside the sterilizer and prevent proper steam penetration of devices in the load and would compromise sterility. To avoid false failures, always run the B-D test in a warm sterilizer. Heat the sterilizer by running a shortened, empty-chamber cycle. Place the test pack in an empty sterilizer on the bottom shelf, over the drain. The cycle is run as specified by the sterilizer manufacturer. The recommended exposure time is 3.5 to 4 minutes. The exposure time should never exceed 4 minutes at 134°C (273°F). If longer exposure times are used, the test should be considered invalid and the results meaningless; even an extra minute could affect the results.[21] After processing the B-D test pack, the indicator sheet inside will show

Table 5
Routine sterilizer efficacy testing of flash sterilization processes
Run an empty cycle in a dynamic air-removal (prevacuum) sterilizer to preheat it and purge air from the lines
Place a Bowie-Dick (B-D) test pack horizontally in the front, bottom section of the sterilizer rack, near the door over the drain, but not on the floor unless recommended by the B-D manufacturer if it is a dynamic air-removal (prevacuum) sterilizer
Run the sterilizer for 3.5–4 min at 132–135°C
Read the physical monitors and initial the printout
Interpret the B-D indicator sheet according to the manufacturer's guide and, if there is no problem, begin daily sterilization routine
Choose the appropriate PCD (BI challenge test pack) for each sterilization mode or cycle and tray configuration used daily (**Table 6**)
Label the PCD (BI challenge test pack) with the appropriate sterilizer lot and load information
Place 1 or more BIs and 1 or more CIs in the areas of the tray configurations determined to create the greatest challenge to air removal and sterilant penetration
Place the PCD (BI challenge test pack) in an empty sterilizer on the bottom rack near the drain in the area least favorable to sterilization according to the manufacturer's instructions. Performing the test in an empty chamber minimizes heating time on spore kill that occurs when a heavy metal mass is in the load
Run the load according to the sterilizer manufacturer's instructions
Read the physical monitors, verify, and initial the printout
On completion of the cycle, cool the BI, PCD, and BIs according to the manufacturer's instructions
Remove CIs from the PCD and record the results following the manufacturer's instructions for interpretation
Incubate the test BIs and a control BI from the same lot that has not been exposed to the sterilant in the same autoreader or incubator
Read and record the test and control results on completion of the incubation stage[33]

a uniform color change to pass, as indicated by the manufacturer's interpretation guide. The B-D test does not test sterilization; it tests only air removal. Results are read and recorded on removal of the test pack.

ROUTINE STERILIZATION MONITORING WITH BIS

BIs used for steam sterilization are typically supplied as commercially prepared ampoules that consist of highly resistant live spores accompanied by incubation media. The BIs should consist of spores of *Geobacillus stearothermophilus* that comply with ANSI/AAMI/ISO 11138-3:2006 and that are suitable for use in the specific sterilization cycle. Data should be obtained from manufacturers on the reliability, safety, and performance characteristics of their products. Manufacturers of BIs are required to provide written instructions on the storage, handling, use, and microbiological testing of their products. BIs are intended to establish whether the conditions were adequate to achieve sterilization. All BIs should be used in accordance with the BI manufacturer's instructions.[22] BIs provide the only devices for sterilization process monitoring that provide a direct measure of the lethality of the sterilization process. BIs must be incubated for various periods of time (depending on the specific product) until it is determined whether the microorganisms grow (ie, they survived the sterilization process) or fail to grow (ie, they were killed by the sterilization process).

Each type of sterilizer cycle (gravity displacement or dynamic air removal [prevacuum]) and each type of tray configuration used in flash sterilization should be tested with a BI PCD as shown in **Table 6**. The same type of tray to be routinely processed through the flash sterilizer should be selected to serve as the PCD (BI challenge test tray). Each type of tray configuration in routine use for flash sterilization should be tested separately. One or more BIs and CIs should be placed in the empty tray configuration to be tested. The PCD (BI challenge test tray) should be of appropriate size for the sterilizer being tested. The BIs and CIs should be located in the most difficult-to-sterilize portion of the PCD. For perforated mesh-bottom, open surgical trays, single-wrapped surgical trays, and protective organizing cases, the most difficult-to-sterilize area is the area nearest the sterilizer drain. In each rigid sterilization container system to be tested, BIs and CIs should be placed strategically alongside each other at locations that present the greatest challenge to air evacuation and sterilant penetration. Particularly in gravity-displacement steam sterilizers, the corners of the container system and the underside of the lid, away from the filters, are the likeliest locations for air pockets. Because the areas of greatest challenge to steam penetration and air removal vary from one rigid sterilization container system to another, the container manufacturer should be consulted for appropriate monitoring locations and placement of CIs and BIs. The PCD (BI challenge test tray) should be placed on the bottom shelf of an empty sterilizer because, for flash sterilization, this configuration is a more rigorous biologic challenge to sterilizer performance than a filled chamber. Performing the test in an empty chamber minimizes heating time (because there is little metal mass to absorb the heat) and, therefore, minimizes the lethality of the process and creates a greater challenge to the BI. Placement near the drain generally ensures that the PCD is in the coolest portion of the chamber, but the sterilizer manufacturer is best able to advise the user on the cold point.[23] Considering the different types of sterilizer cycles and the high volume in large ORs, placing a BI in every load is good judgment. Monitoring every load ensures that any set containing an implant (screw, plate, wire, and so forth) will not inadvertently be released without a BI having been run with the load. It makes it easier to track the implant back to the patient.

Table 6
BI PCDs[a] for different cycle/tray configurations for routine testing of flash sterilization cycle[b]

Type of Cycle	Tray Configuration Tested Separately	BI PCD Placed in Empty Tray
Gravity displacement	Perforated, mesh-bottomed, open surgical tray	BI and CI in open, perforated, mesh-bottom surgical tray
Gravity displacement	Rigid sterilization container system	BIs and CIs should be placed strategically alongside each other at locations that present the greatest challenge to air evacuation and sterilant penetration
Gravity displacement	Protective organizing case	BIs and CIs should be placed strategically alongside each other at locations that present the greatest challenge to air evacuation and sterilant penetration
Dynamic air removal (prevacuum)	Perforated, mesh-bottomed, open surgical tray	BI and CI in open, perforated, mesh-bottom surgical tray
Dynamic air removal (prevacuum)	Rigid sterilization container	BIs and CIs should be placed strategically alongside each other at locations that present the greatest challenge to air evacuation and sterilant penetration
Dynamic air removal (prevacuum)	Protective organizing case	BIs and CIs should be placed strategically alongside each other at locations that present the greatest challenge to air evacuation and sterilant penetration
Dynamic air removal (prevacuum)	Single-wrapped surgical tray	BIs and CIs should be placed strategically alongside each other at locations that present the greatest challenge to air evacuation and sterilant penetration

[a] Commercially available BI PCDs may be used if designed for the type of cycle, time, and temperature, and if they create a challenge that is equal to or greater then the type of tray configuration.
[b] Sterilization times determined by medical device, container, and sterilizer manufacturer. Recommend exposure time is 3.5–4 minutes. The exposure time should never exceed 4 minutes at 134°C. If longer exposure times are used, the test should be considered invalid and the results meaningless; even an extra minute could affect the results.
From AAMI ST79:2006:A2:2009. Comprehensive guide to steam sterilization and sterility assurance in health care facilities. Arlington (VA): Association for the Advancement of Medical Instrumentation, 2006:A2:2009:10.7.4.1. p. 92 and 10.10.3.2.2. p. 104–5; with permission.

ROUTINE STERILIZATION MONITORING WITH CIS

CIs are designed to respond with a chemical or physical change to 1 or more of the physical conditions within the sterilizing chamber and they are not interchangeable. CIs assist in the detection of potential sterilization failures that could result from incorrect packaging, incorrect loading of the sterilizer, or malfunctions of the sterilizer. An internal CI should be used within each package, tray, or rigid sterilization container system to be sterilized to provide immediate results indicating whether the conditions for sterilization were met. The CI should be placed in that area of the package, tray, or containment device (rigid sterilization container system, instrument case, cassette, or organizing tray) considered to be least accessible to steam penetration; for a containment device, the manufacturer's instructions for placement of the CI should be consulted. The CI is retrieved at the time of use and is interpreted by the user. The pass response of a CI does not prove that the item monitored by the indicator is sterile. The use of CIs is part of an effective quality assurance program that should be used in conjunction with physical monitors and BIs to establish the efficacy of the sterilization process. All CIs should be used in accordance with the CI manufacturer's instructions. CIs should be used on the outside and inside of every item sterilized.

There are 6 classes of CIs intended for specific use:

- Class 1. Process indicators are for use with individual units (eg, packs, containers) to indicate that the unit has been exposed to the sterilization process and to distinguish between processed and unprocessed units. These indicators are also referred to as external CIs placed on the outside of every package and container to be sterilized. Class 1 indicators are usually in the form of tape or a label on the outside of the item. When removing items from the sterilizer, items are checked for the expected change of the indicator. For flash sterilization, a CI should be affixed to the outside of the container. It is the first indicator checked before a sterile item is opened because it is on the outside of a container or package. It provides the first warning sign if it did not reach the expected parameters (usually change of color in the tape or indicator). A class 1 Indicator is the first visible sign (change in color) that the item has been exposed to the sterilant. If the indicator did not reach the expected change in color or indicator movement, it is the first warning signal to not use the item and investigate further as to why the parameters were not reached. It does not provide any indication of whether the exposure time or temperature met the required parameters
- Class 2. (Bowie-Dick test indicator) A chemical indicator designed for use in a specific test procedure (eg, the Bowie-Dick test is used to determine if air removal has been adequate in the steam sterilization process)
- Class 3. Single-variable indicators are designed to react to one of the critical variables and are intended to indicate exposure to a sterilization process. They usually measure temperature or time
- Class 4. Multivariable indicators are designed to react to 2 or more of the critical variables and are intended to indicate exposure to a sterilization process. They usually measure temperature and time
- Class 5. Integrating indicators are designed to react to all critical variables, with the stated values having been generated to be equivalent to, or exceed, the performance requirements given in the ISO 11138 series for BIs. They measure all the cycle parameters necessary for SAL 10-6 (the standard for sterilization of medical devices). An integrating indicator provides more information than other types of CIs. AORN recommends that a class 5 integrating indicator should be used on the inside of each tray or container to be sterilized. It should be placed in an area within the tray or container that has been determined to be the least accessible to steam contact. Suggested placements are:
  in the geometric center of a wrapped pack or tray
  in 2 opposite corners of the inner baskets of containers
  in 2 opposite corners on every level of multilevel wrapped sets.

The container manufacturer should also be consulted to determine the most challenging location within the container.[24]

- Class 6. Emulating indicators are cycle verification indicators designed to react to all critical variables of specified sterilization cycles, with the stated values having been generated from the critical variables of the specific sterilization process.[25]

CIs are not interchangeable. They give you different information, and they all have value. No indicator can guarantee the sterility of a product and, no matter what happens with these indicators, they do not guarantee that the items in the sterilization load have become sterile. Indicators are guides that assist in recognizing whether items have been exposed to a sterilization process. They are not a guarantee that the items are sterile; it is the process of decontamination, thorough cleaning, package/container assembly, sterilization, and quality monitoring that determines whether items are sterile.[26] **Table 7** lists the types and applications for use of sterilization monitoring devices.

IMPLANTS

The FDA's definition of an implant is a device that is placed into a surgically or naturally formed body cavity with the intention of remaining there for a period of 30 days or more. Implantable devices should never be flash sterilized per recommendations from CDC, AAMI, AORN, and The Joint Commission. Implants remain in the body, and infections that involve them are significantly more difficult to treat and often require surgical intervention to resolve the infection by removing the implant. Flash sterilization should not be used for implantable devices except in cases of emergency when no other option is available. Implants are foreign bodies and they increase the risk of SSI.[27]

All plantable devices require documentation of cycle information and monitoring results that should be maintained in a log (electronic or manual) to provide tracking of the flashed items to the individual patient for at least 1 year after they have been implanted. Careful planning, appropriate packaging, and inventory management in cooperation with suppliers can minimize the need to flash sterilize implantable medical devices. In an emergency, when flash sterilization of an implant is unavoidable, a rapid-action BI with a class 5 chemical integrating indicator should be run with the load. The BI monitoring is necessary to provide optimal sterility assurance providing additional information about the critical parameters of the sterilization process. The implant should be quarantined on the back table and should not be implanted until the rapid-action BI provides a negative result. If the implant is used before the BI results are known and the BI is later determined to have a positive result, the surgeon and infection prevention professional should be notified as soon as the results are known. If the implant is not used, it cannot be saved as sterile for future use. Resterilization of the device is required if the implant is to be used later.[4]

RELEASE CRITERIA FOR IMPLANTS

The decision to release a load should be made by an experienced, knowledgeable person at the conclusion of the sterilization cycle. The sterilizer operator should review the physical monitors (eg, printout) and the results of other indicators that have been used to monitor the sterilization process. The load should be quarantined until the results of the BI testing are available and show negative results.[28]

Table 7
Types and applications for use of sterilization monitoring devices

Monitor	Frequency of Use	Application (Release of Sterilizer, Package, Load)
Physical monitors		
Time, temperature, and pressure recorders, displays, digital printouts, and gauges	Should be used for every load of every sterilizer	Part of load release criteria
Chemical Indicators (CIs)		
External CIs Class 1 (process indicators)	Should be used on outside of every package	Part of load and package release criteria
B-D-type indicators Class 2 (B-D)	For routine sterilizer testing (dynamic air-removal [prevacuum] sterilizers only), should be run, within a test pack, each day in an empty sterilizer before the first processed load For sterilizer qualification testing (dynamic air-removal sterilizers only), should be run, within a test pack, after sterilizer installation, relocation, malfunction, and major repairs and after sterilization process failures; test should be run 3 times consecutively in an empty chamber after BI tests	Test of sterilizer for efficacy of air removal and steam penetration; part of release criteria for using sterilizer for the day Part of release criteria for placing sterilizer into service after qualification testing
Internal CIs	Should be used inside each package Should be used in periodic product quality assurance testing	Part of package release criteria at use site Part of release criteria for changes made to routinely sterilized items, load configuration, or packaging Release criteria should include BI results
Class 3 (single-variable indicator) Class 4 (multivariable indicator)	May be used to meet internal CI recommendation	Part of package release criteria at use site; Not to be used for release of loads

Class 5 (integrating indicator)	May be used to meet internal CI recommendation Within a PCD,[a] may be used to monitor nonimplant sterilizer loads Within a PCD, should be used to monitor each sterilizer load containing implants. The PCD should also contain a BI	Part of package release criteria at use site Part of load release criteria for nonimplant loads Part of release criteria for loads containing implants. Except in emergencies, implants should be quarantined until BI results are known
BIs	Within a PCD, may be used to monitor nonimplant loads Within a PCD, should be used in every load containing implants The PCD should also contain a class 5 integrating indicator	Part of load release criteria Part of release criteria for loads containing implants Except in emergencies, implants should be quarantined until BI results are known
BIs	Within a PCD, should be used weekly, and preferably daily (each day the sterilizer is used), routine sterilizer efficacy testing. (The PCD may also contain a CI.) Should be run in a full load for wrapped items; for table-top sterilization, should be run in a fully loaded chamber; for flash sterilization, should be run in an empty chamber Within a PCD, should be used for sterilizer qualification testing (after sterilizer installation, relocation, malfunction, major repairs, sterilization process failures). The PCD may also contain a CI. Tests should be run 3 times consecutively in an empty chamber, except for table-top sterilizers, for which the test should be run 3 times consecutively in a full load Should be used for periodic product quality assurance testing	Part of sterilizer/load release and recall criteria Part of release criteria for placing sterilizer into service after qualification testing Part of release criteria for changes made to routinely sterilized items, load configuration, or packaging

[a] PCDs are designed to constitute a defined resistance to a sterilization process and are used to assess the performance of the process.

From Association for the Advancement of Medical Instrumentation. Comprehensive guide to steam sterilization and sterility assurance in health care facilities. ANSI/AAMI ST79: 2006/A2:2009. p. 82. Section of Table 7; with permission.

A BI PCD containing a class 5 integrating CI should be used in each load containing an implant. To improve patient safety, the load should be quarantined until the BI is negative. The following monitoring should be done:

- Physically monitor each load
- Label every container with an external process indicator
- Place an internal CI inside each container
- Monitor with a PCD containing a BI and a class 5 integrating CI
- Evaluate all quality control measures and data at the conclusion of the sterilization cycle (this should be done by an experienced, knowledgeable person)
- Quarantine the implant until BI is negative
- Release loads only if the criteria for release are present.[29]

When documented medical exceptions dictate (eg, the need for trauma-related orthopedic screw-plate sets), it could be necessary to release an implantable device before the BI results are known. In this case, the release of the device before the BI results are known should be documented; the BI result obtained later should also be documented. The documentation process is particularly important when implants are flash sterilized. AAMI recommends a dedicated exception form to facilitate detailed documentation of premature release of an implant and it is critical that this record be fully traceable to the patient (**Table 8** shows a sample exception form and **Table 9** gives an example of documentation of a premature release implant

---

Table 8
Exception form for premature release of implantable device/tray

NOTE: In a documented emergency situation, implantable devices will be released from quarantine in CS/SPD without a biological monitor result. This form should accompany the implant to the Operating Room. OR personnel should complete this form and return it to CS/SPD within 24 hours.

PLEASE COMPLETE ALL INFORMATION

Date:	Time:	Shift:
Person completing report in CS/SPD:		
List the implantable devices/trays prematurely released to the OR:		
OR person requesting premature release of devices:		

Operating Room Portion of Report	
Date of Procedure:	Time of Procedure:
Patient Name/Sticker:	Surgeon Name:
Reason premature release was needed:	
What could have prevented premature release of this device/tray?	
Name of person completing report:	
Date report completed:	Date form returned to CS/SPD:

Table 9
Example of documentation of premature release of implants

Date	Description of Implant	Time Sterilized	Sterilizer #	Load #	Date/time BI in Incubator	Date/time BI Results	Early Release (Y/N)	Date/time Released to OR	Released by (Full Name)

log). Releasing implants before the BI results are known is unacceptable and should be the exception, not the rule. Emergency situations should be defined in written guidance developed in consultation with an infection-prevention professional, the surgeon, and risk management. Steps should be taken to reduce the frequency of emergency release of implantable items. For example, ongoing periodic reviews of the exception forms and implant logs could reveal consistent patterns of events that are causing emergency release and that could be corrected. Patient safety could be adversely affected by the implantation of a nonsterile device. The sterilization of implantables should be closely monitored and each load containing implants should be quarantined until it is verified that BI testing has yielded negative results. In defined emergency situations in which the quarantine of implants cannot be maintained, breaking of the quarantine is allowed for documented medical exceptions in accordance with facility policies and procedures. Flash sterilization should not be used as a substitute for sufficient instrument inventory resulting from late delivery of loaner instruments. All loaner instruments should be ordered in a timely matter to prevent any flash sterilization.

STAFF EDUCATION AND TRAINING

Managers must ensure that staff members are adequately trained to correctly, effectively, and consistently perform the tasks of flash sterilization. Staff training and competency are critical to reprocessing, and recommendations include the following:

- Providing comprehensive and intensive training for all reprocessing staff
- Supervising work until competency is documented
- Validating competency by testing at hiring and annually
- Reviewing instructions regularly to make sure staff comply with the literature and manufacturers' instructions
- Conducting real-time audits.

Sterilization-specific education and competency assessment of personnel should encompass all sterilization methodologies in use in the organization, to include the following:

- Operation and maintenance of sterilization equipment
- Selection and monitoring of sterilization cycles
- Use of chemical, biologic, and physical monitoring measures
- Documentation requirements.

Education should address, but not be limited to:

- Orientation programs to equipment and work area
- Infection-control policy and procedure, including exposure plans
- Potential hazards in the environment and methods of hazard protection
- Safe ergonomic practices
- Use and location of material safety data sheets (MSDS).[4]

It is critical that personnel are knowledgeable and competent, especially in the decontamination and cleaning processes. Ongoing education and competency validation of perioperative personnel facilitates the development of knowledge, skills, and attitudes that affect patient and worker safety. Personnel should receive initial education on the following:

- Decontamination methods
- Preparation of instruments and equipment for sterilization

- Selection of cleaning agents and methods
- Proper use of cleaning agents, including an understanding of specific applications, appropriate dilution, and special precautions
- Decontamination of specific instruments and equipment used within the practice setting
- Procedures for decontamination of instruments contaminated with prions and the effectiveness of various methods of deactivation
- Personal protection required during instrument processing
- Exposure risk associated with chemical cleaning agents.

Workers have the right to know the hazards that exist in the workplace and OSHA requires that employers provide this information.[12] Understanding procedures involved in cleaning each type of instrument is necessary to provide the foundation for compliance with procedures. Personnel should receive education on:

- New instruments and equipment
- New cleaning agents and methods
- New procedures.

Administrative personnel should validate the competencies of personnel participating in decontamination of surgical instruments. The validation of competencies should include all types of instruments that the individual is authorized to reprocess. Validation of competencies provides an indication that personnel are able to appropriately perform decontamination procedures.[9]

LOANER INSTRUMENTATION

Implementation of tracking and quality controls and procedures are necessary to manage instrumentation and implants brought in from outside organizations and companies. The systematic management of loaner instrumentation reduces loss and ensures proper decontamination and sterilization through increased communication and accountability. Guidelines for managing and processing loaner instrumentation are shown in **Table 10**.

DOCUMENTATION/RECORDING

Cycle information and monitoring results of all items that are flash sterilized should be documented and maintained in a log (electronic or manual) to provide tracking of the flashed items to the individual patient. Documentation allows every load of sterilized items used on patients to be traced, so careful monitoring of sterilizers is a must. After each load, the recording device must be checked to verify that conditions for sterilization were met. Sterilization records should include the following information on each load, including the item(s) processed:

- Patient receiving the item
- Cycle parameters used (eg, temperature, duration of cycle)
- Date and time the cycle is run
- Operator information
- Reason for flash sterilization.[4]

Table 11 is a sample of a daily flash sterilization record that includes information to track the flash-sterilized device back to the patient. Accurate and complete records are required for process verification and can be used in sterilizer malfunction analyses.

Table 10
Loaner instrumentation process guidelines

Request loaner instrumentation or implant at the time patient is scheduled for surgery
    Specify quantities of loaner items and estimated time of use and return
    State restocking requirements to circumvent any need for flash sterilization

Obtain manufacturers' written instruction for instrument care, cleaning, assembly, and sterilization
Deliver instrumentation in a timely manner to avoid any flash sterilization
Receive loaner items, including a detailed inventory list, at a time designated by the facility to complete all steps of the sterilization process and results of the BI before the scheduled surgery time
Consider all loaner instruments to be contaminated and to be delivered directly to the decontamination area for processing
Clean, decontaminate, and sterilize borrowed instrumentation in a manner consistent with AORN's "recommended practices for cleaning and care of surgical instruments and powered equipment" and the standards of AAMI before sterilization
Follow the same sterilization process for newly manufactured loaner items to remove bioburden and substances (eg, oils, greases, particles) remaining on the item from the manufacturing process
Remove packaging from instrumentation previously sterilized from another facility and follow the same sterilization process
Remove instrumentation from transport/shipping containers (these may have high microbial contamination from environmental exposures during transport) before entering the SPD or areas of the surgical suite
Inspect containers for integrity and function and visually inspect instruments or implants for damage
Inventory and document the type and quantity of loaner items received
Transport processed instrumentation to the point of use (operative/invasive area) carefully to avoid comprising the packaging or containers
Return items after use to the SPD following the procedure for decontamination, processing, inventory, and return to the health care industry representative
Maintain historical records of all transactions

From AORN standards and recommended practices for sterilization in the perioperative practice setting. In: Perioperative standards, recommended practices. Denver (CO): AORN, Inc; 2009. p. 658–9; with permission.

Documentation establishes accountability. The record should be placed on a clip board and attached to each sterilizer that is used for flash sterilization. The information obtained from the documentation process can be used to determine factors or trends that lead to flash sterilization and to identify and implement procedures to prevent further occurrences.

PRODUCT IDENTIFICATION AND TRACEABILITY

Physical gauges, such as time, temperature, and pressure, should be recorded for each sterilizer cycle. CIs should be used on the inside and outside of every processed package. Perioperative personnel should review and initial sterilizer charts and print-outs after each cycle and before opening the door. For flash sterilization, labels with lot numbers are not used; however, a lot number should be assigned to each flash

Table 11

DAILY FLASH STERILIZATION RECORD

Date:_____   Autoclave #_____

Time:	OR #	Patient label	Reason for FLASH? ☐ Not enough/incorrect instruments ☐ Contaminated – no replacement ☐ Vendor–arrived <4^0 to start time ☐ Surgeon personal Instruments ☐ Other_____
Gravity	Prevac		
270° 3 min	270° 3 min		
270° 10 min	270° 4 min	Surgeon Name & Item Description	Started By (Initials): _____ Implant? Y / N BI Run? Y / N Removed By (Initials): _____ CI Indicator Verified: Y / N
Cycle #			
Time:	OR #	Patient label	Reason for FLASH? ☐ Not enough/incorrect instruments ☐ Contaminated – no replacement ☐ Vendor–arrived <4^0 to start time ☐ Surgeon personal Instruments ☐ Other_____
Gravity	Prevac		
270° 3 min	270° 3 min		
270° 10 min	270° 4 min	Surgeon Name & Item Description	Started By (Initials): _____ Implant? Y / N BI Run? Y / N Removed By (Initials): _____ CI Indicator Verified: Y / N
Cycle #			
Time:	OR #	Patient Label	Reason for FLASH? ☐ Not enough/incorrect instruments ☐ Contaminated – no replacement ☐ Vendor–arrived <4^0 to start time ☐ Surgeon personal Instruments ☐ Other_____
Gravity	Prevac		
270° 3 min	270° 3 min		
270° 10 min	270° 4 min	Surgeon Name & Item Description	Started By (Initials): _____ Implant? Y / N BI Run? Y / N Removed By (Initials): _____ CI Indicator Verified: Y / N
Cycle #			
Time:	OR #	Patient Label	Reason for FLASH? ☐ Not enough/incorrect instruments ☐ Contaminated – no replacement ☐ Vendor–arrived <4^0 to start time ☐ Surgeon personal Instruments ☐ Other_____
Gravity	Prevac		
270° 3 min	270° 3 min		
270° 10 min	270° 4 min	Surgeon Name & Item Description	Started By (Initials): _____ Implant? Y / N BI Run? Y / N Removed By (Initials): _____ CI Indicator Verified: Y / N
Cycle #			
Time:	OR #	Patient Label	Reason for FLASH? ☐ Not enough/incorrect instruments ☐ Contaminated – no replacement ☐ Vendor–arrived <4^0 to start time ☐ Surgeon personal Instruments ☐ Other_____
Gravity	Prevac		
270° 3 min	270° 3 min		
270° 10 min	270° 4 min	Surgeon Name & Item Description	Started By (Initials): _____ Implant? Y / N BI Run? Y / N Removed By (Initials): _____ CI Indicator Verified: Y / N
Cycle #			

*BI – Biological Indicator
*CI – Chemical Indicator

sterilization load and a load record should be generated for each sterilization cycle. The load record should document the following:

- Assigned lot number, including sterilizer identification and cycle number
- General contents of the load

- Duration and temperature of the exposed phase of the cycle
- The signature or other identification of the operator
- Date and time of the cycle.[30]

Policy and procedure manuals on flash sterilization should be written, reviewed annually, and available for reference. Staff should be knowledgeable and attend annual reviews on infection prevention and control: proper hand washing, scrub attire, PPE, blood-borne pathogens standards, HAI, and principles of asepsis.[31] Standardization and consistency in following the steps of the flash sterilization process are key to ensuring that devices are sterile, thus decreasing the patient's risk of an SSI. Policies and procedures establish authority, responsibility, and accountability, and serve as operational guidelines. They also assist in the development of continuous quality-improvement activities.

QUALITY CONTROL

AORN recommends that a quality control program should be established and maintained that enhances personnel performance and monitors sterilization efficacy to promote patient and employee safety.[4] Quality monitoring of steam sterilization includes, but is not limited to, the use of physical-equipment, chemical, and biologic monitors; sterilizer efficacy; load monitoring and release; product testing ;and product recall management. Verification of the flash sterilization process of instruments used during the operative/invasive procedure is part of the perioperative nurse's responsibility. Daily audits should be performed on flash sterilization records following these guidelines:

- Audit daily sterilization records for correct documentation; this should be 100%
- Audit previous day's record (daily)
- Report discrepancies to manager and staff
- Alert infection prevention professional and committees
- Educate staff (all on same page) to be prepared when questioned by regulatory agencies.

Quality control programs that enhance personnel performance and monitor sterilization efficacy are established to promote patient and employee safety. Monitoring the sterilization process allows results to be compared with a predetermined level of quality. Reviewing the findings provides a method of identifying problems and trends to change and improve practice. A list of sterilization resources and references is given in **Table 12** to assist with quality management programs.

THE JOINT COMMISSION

The Joint Commission is focusing on the process necessary for optimal patient outcomes. Dr Robert Wise, MD, vice president of standards at The Joint Commission, stated that "We will move away from focusing simply on the method of steam sterilization to looking at the process in a broader and more rigorous way; from the time the instruments leave the OR to their return." Joint Commission surveyors will focus on all of the critical steps and the integrity of the sterilization process.

Among other activities, surveyors will:

- Observe instruments from the time they leave one OR to when they are returned to the next

Table 12
Sterilization resources/references

Organization	Address	Telephone	Web site
AAMI	1110 N Glebe Rd, Suite 220, Arlington, VA 22201-4795	703 525 4890	www.aami.org.
AORN	2170 S Parker Rd, Suite 300, Denver, CO 80231-5711	303 755 6300 or 800 755 AORN	www.aorn.org
International Association of Healthcare Central Service Material Management (IAHCSMM)	213 W Institute Pl, Suite 307, Chicago, IL 60610-9432	800 962 8274	www.iahcsmm.org
CDC	1600 Clifton Road, Atlanta, GA 30333	404 639 3534 or 800 311 3435	www.cdc.gov
OSHA	200 Constitution Avenue, NW, Washington, DC 2021	202 523 7725	www.osha.gov
Center for Medicare & Medicaid Services (CMS)	7500 Security Boulevard, Baltimore, MD 21244-1850	877 267 2323	www.cms.gov
The Joint Commission (TJC)	One Renaissance Boulevard, Oakbrook Terrace, IL 60181	630 792 5000	www. jointcommission. org
American Society of Cataract and Refractive Surgery (ASCRS)	4000 Legato Road Ste 700, Fairfax, VA 22033	703 591 2220	www.ascrs.org

- Ask health care workers to provide the manufacturers' instructions for instrument sterilization, and to describe and demonstrate how instruments are being cleaned and decontaminated according to those written instructions
- Observe the cleaning of instruments. Rinsing is rarely enough to properly remove soil from instruments; meticulous cleaning is needed
- Verify that staff members are wearing appropriate PPE
- Observe the sterilization process. The surveyor will ask for the manufacturer's instructions for the sterilizer, wrapping or packing, and the instruments
- Review sterilization logs. Surveyors will ask about parametric, CIs and BIs
- Observe the return of instruments to the sterile field and verify that they are being protected from recontamination
- View the entire Steam Sterilization–Update on the Joint Commission's Position.[32]

Experts in sterilization representing AAMI and AORN consider some aspects of the update to be confusing. One issue is the description of flash sterilization as a cycle of "3 minutes at 270°F at 27 to 28 lbs of pressure." The description does not refer to dry time, or differentiate between gravity and prevacuum cycles, or mention that flash-sterilized items are intended for immediate use. Reconciling manufacturers' instructions is another concern. It is not always possible to reconcile instructions for sets that require extended cycles, which have become increasingly common. AORN discussed sterilization issues with the Joint Commission in 2009 but was not asked to review or comment on the update before it was released. Further discussions on how to clarify these statements are ongoing between the sterilization experts and the Joint Commission.[33]

SUMMARY

The process of flash sterilization continues to evolve focusing on what is needed to guarantee that flash sterilization is safe, effective and will ultimately ensure patient safety and reduce SSIs. In order to increase the probability that the item is safe for patient use, the process should include the manufacturers' instructions (many recommending longer cycles for devices), strict cleaning procedures, the use of closed containers and stringent documentation to assist in tracing the entire flash sterilization process. Because of the changes, today's practice is more complex with the necessity for increased knowledge and staff competencies of the entire sterilization process. The imperative that effective cleaning of devices must precede sterilization is well established. When selecting the parameters for flash sterilization the type of cycle (gravity or dynamic air-removal [prevacuum]) and the correct temperature and time all depend on the items being flash sterilized. The following table summarizes cycle, temperature and time for specific items.

Cycle Type	Dynamic Air Removal (Prevacuum)	Gravity
Temperature	270° F–275° F (132° C–135° C)	270° F–275° F (132° C–135° C)
Time (min)	3 minutes Metal, nonporous, no lumen items	3 minutes Metal, nonporous, no lumen items
Time (min)	4 minutes Metal, porous, w/lumen items	10 minutes Metal, porous, w/lumen items

The way that regulatory agencies review or assess a facility's process for flash sterilization is also changing. Sterilization processes are assessed to ensure that they achieve the most important end: delivering safe products for patients. Because of the increased incidences of SSIs and HAIs, it is imperative that all steps of the sterilization process be followed consistently and conscientiously. When a facility can ensure that all of the critical steps are met and correct practices according to ANSI/AAIM, AORN, CDC, HICPAC, and OSHA are being followed, then the facility can be confident of satisfying the regulatory agencies.

When done correctly, flash sterilization is a safe and effective process for the sterilization of instruments intended for immediate use during operative/invasive procedures. But the use of flash sterilization should be kept to a minimum. Demands for patient safety and infection prevention highlight the need to have effective flash sterilization policies and procedures in place to achieve effective outcomes. To minimize infection risks, perioperative managers should review and audit current practices and implement a workable, continuous, quality-improvement program.

REFERENCES

1. Mitchell S. Practicing the complete sterilization process. AORN Connections 2009;5(1):1–2.
2. Perkins J. Principles and methods of sterilization in health sciences. Springfield (IL): Charles C Thomas; 1982.

3. ANSI/AAMI ST79:2006A2:2009 Comprehensive guide to steam sterilization and sterility assurance in health care facilities. Arlington (VA): Association for the Advancement of Medical Instrumentation; 2006. A2:2009:2.50.

4. AORN standards and recommended practices for sterilization in the perioperative practice setting. In: Perioperative standards, recommended practices. Denver (CO): AORN, Inc; 2009. p. 647–70.

5. Hancock CO. Steam sterilization: sterilizer operation. In: Reichert M, Young JH, editors. Sterilization technology for the healthcare facility. 2nd edition. Gaithersburg (MD): Aspen Publications; 1997. p. 134–45.

6. Atherton M, Corriher J, Leonard Y, et al. Evaluating use of flash sterilization in the OR. AORN J 2006;83(3):672–80.

7. Spry C. Sterilization and infection control: the importance of cleaning in earnest. OR Manager 2008;24(5):20–2.

8. US Department of Labor, Occupational Safety and Health Administration. Bloodborne pathogens. 26CFR 1910.1030. Available at: http://www.osha.gov/pls/oshaweb/owadisp.show_document?p_table=STANDARDS&p_id=10051. Accessed August 20, 2009.

9. AORN standards and recommended practices for cleaning and care of surgical instruments and power equipment. In: Perioperative standards, recommended practices. Denver (CO): AORN, Inc; 2009. p. 611–35.

10. ANSI/AAMI ST79:2006:A2:2009 Comprehensive guide to steam sterilization and sterility assurance in health care facilities. Arlington (VA): Association for the Advancement of Medical Instrumentation; 2006. A2:2009: 7.1.

11. Centers for Disease Control and Prevention. Guideline for hand hygiene in healthcare settings. Available at: http://www.cdc.gov/mmwr/preview/mmwrhtml/rr5116a1.htm. Accessed August 21, 2009.

12. Occupational Safety and Health Administration. Hazard communication: OSHA standards. Available at: http://osha.gov/SLTC/hazardcommunications/standards.html. Accessed August 20, 2009.

13. ANSI/AAMI ST79:2006:A2:2009 Comprehensive guide to steam sterilization and sterility assurance in health care facilities. Arlington (VA): Association for the Advancement of Medical Instrumentation; 2006. A2:2009: 7.5.5.

14. Kutty PK, Forster TS, Wood-Koob C, et al. Multistate outbreak of toxic anterior segment syndrome. J Cataract Refract Surg 2008;34(4):585–90.

15. Mamalis N, Edelhauser HF, Dawson DG, et al. Toxic anterior segment syndrome. J Cataract Refract Surg 2006;32:324–33.

16. Kim JH. Intraocular inflammation of denatured viscoelastic substance in cases of cataract extraction and lens implantation. J Cataract Refract Surg 1987;13:537–42.

17. ANSI/AAMI ST79:2006:A2:2009 Comprehensive guide to steam sterilization and sterility assurance in health care facilities. Arlington (VA): Association for the Advancement of Medical Instrumentation; 2006. A2:2009:8.8.3,4,5.

18. Steris Study Guide. The hot issues of flash sterilization: study guide # 1. Available at: http://www.steris.com/healthcare/ser_edu_study.cfm. Accessed September 17, 2009.

19. ANSI/AAMI ST79:2006:A2:2009 Comprehensive guide to steam sterilization and sterility assurance in health care facilities. Arlington (VA): Association for the Advancement of Medical Instrumentation; 2006. A2:2009:8.8.5.

20. ANSI/AAMI ST79:2006:A2:2009 Comprehensive guide to steam sterilization and sterility assurance in health care facilities. Arlington (VA): Association for the Advancement of Medical Instrumentation; 2006. A2:2009:10.5.4.

21. ANSI/AAMI ST79:2006:A2:2009 Comprehensive guide to steam sterilization and sterility assurance in health care facilities. Arlington (VA): Association for the Advancement of Medical Instrumentation; 2006. A2:2009:10.7.6.4.

22. ANSI/AAMI ST79:2006:A2:2009 Comprehensive guide to steam sterilization and sterility assurance in health care facilities. Arlington (VA): Association for the Advancement of Medical Instrumentation; 2006. A2:2009:10.5.3.1.

23. ANSI/AAMI ST79:2006:A2:2009 Comprehensive guide to steam sterilization and sterility assurance in health care facilities. Arlington (VA): Association for the Advancement of Medical Instrumentation; 2006. A2:2009:10.7.4.1 & 1010.2.2.1.

24. AORN standards and recommended practices for selection and use of packaging systems for sterilization. In: Perioperative standards, recommended practices. Denver (CO): AORN, Inc; 2009. p. 637–46.

25. ANSI/AAMI ST79:2006:A2:2009 Comprehensive guide to steam sterilization and sterility assurance in health care facilities. Arlington (VA): Association for the Advancement of Medical Instrumentation; 2006. A2:2009:10.5.2.1.

26. Spry C. Brushing up on use of chemical indicators. OR Manager Inc 2007;23(6): 20–2.

27. Mangram AJ, Horan TC, Pearson ML, et al. Guideline for prevention of surgical site infection, 1999. Infect Control Hosp Epidemiol 1999;20(4):250–78. Available at: http://www.cdc.gov/ncidod/dhqp/pdf/guidelines/SSI.pdf. Accessed July 10, 2009.

28. Centers for Disease Control and Prevention, Healthcare Infection Control Practices Advisory Committee (HICPAC). Guidelines for environmental infection control in health-care facilities. Atlanta (GA): CDC; 2003.

29. Young M. Flash dance. Manag Infec Control 2005;3:62–75.

30. ANSI/AAMI ST79:2006:A2:2009 Comprehensive guide to steam sterilization and sterility assurance in health care facilities. Arlington (VA): Association for the Advancement of Medical Instrumentation; 2006. A2:2009.10.3.1.

31. Seavey R. The need for educated staff in sterile processing-patient safety depends on it. Perioperative Nursing Clinics 2009;4:181–92.

32. The Joint Commission. Steam sterilization–update on the Joint Commission's position. Available at: www.jointcommission.org/Library/WhatsNew/steam_sterilization; June 15, 2009. Accessed August 6, 2009.

33. Seavey R. Flash sterilization: a steaming hot topic. Managing Infection Control 2009;(5):68–80.

Improving the Quality of the Steam Sterilization Process with Appropriate Monitoring Policies and Procedures

Martha L. Young, BS, MS

KEYWORDS

- Perioperative registered nurse • Steam sterilization
- Biological indicators • Chemical indicators

The Association for Perioperative Registered Nurses (AORN) states in the Purpose of the *Recommended Practice for Sterilization in the Perioperative Practice Setting* that "A major responsibility of the perioperative registered nurse is to minimize patient risk for surgical site infection."[1] This goal coincides with the one published on the Association for Professionals in Infection Control and Epidemiology (APIC) Web site, "that every healthcare institution should be working toward a goal of zero healthcare-associated infections."[2]

How does a preoperative registered nurse minimize the risk for surgical site infections when monitoring the steam sterilization process? The answer is by following the recommended practices of the Association for the Advancement of Medical Instrumentation (AAMI), AORN, and Centers for Disease Control and Prevention (CDC), which establish clinical practice.

The *Guideline for Prevention of Surgical Site Infection*, published in 1999 by the CDC states that "Inadequate sterilization of surgical instruments has resulted in SSI outbreaks" and "The importance of routinely monitoring the quality of sterilization procedures has been established."[3] The CDC says this can be accomplished using a biological indicator (BI). The first step is to obtain copies of all of these recommended practices. The next step is to understand the nurse's role in monitoring the

Disclosure: Martha Young is a paid consultant for 3M Infection Prevention Division and a stockholder.
Martha L. Young LLC, SAVVY Sterilization Solutions, 3710 Village Court, MN 55125, USA
E-mail address: marthalyoung1@aol.com

Perioperative Nursing Clinics 5 (2010) 327–345
doi:10.1016/j.cpen.2010.04.005

effectiveness of the steam sterilization process and how it will prevent health care–associated infections.

DEVELOP POLICIES, PROCEDURES, AND STAFF TRAINING

Develop policies and procedures to provide guidelines for maintaining control and determining methods for improvement of the product and process.[4] These policies and procedures should be reviewed and audited for compliance. The written policies and procedures should be based on federal, state, and local recommendations; CDC recommendations; national voluntary standards and recommended practices, such as those of the AAMI and AORN; and device/equipment manufacturer's recommendations.[5]

AORN states that regulatory and accrediting agencies requirements should be included in the policy statement along with the activities that must be completed.[6]

The Joint Commission addresses clinical practice guidelines in the Leadership section of the Hospital Accreditation Standard. The Joint Commission says:

"The hospital considers clinical practice guidelines when designing or improving processes." (LD.04.04.07)[7]

"The hospital provides care, treatment, and services in accordance with licensure requirements, laws and rules, and regulations." (LD.04.01.01)[7]

"Patients with comparable needs receive the same standard of care, treatment, and services throughout the hospital." (LD.04.03.07)[7]

The importance of following evidence-based standards and professional organization guidelines is also stated in the National Patient Safety Goals of the Joint Commission (NPSG.07.05.01) for January 1, 2010 which is to reduce the risk of surgical site infections by aligning policies and practices with evidence-based standards and/or professional organization guidelines.[7]

The AAMI *Comprehensive Guide to Steam Sterilization and Sterility Assurance in Health Care Facilities*, ANSI/AAMI ST79:2006, A1:2008, and A2:2009 states "Education and training decrease the possibility of operator error during preparation and sterilization processing and help ensure that personnel are conversant with the latest data and techniques."[8] Personnel should be trained and monitored to ensure they are following policies and procedures. Critical thinking skills are necessary to understand the science behind the policies and procedures, avoid human errors, and improve the outcome of the sterilization process.

Continuous training and competency assessments help minimize or eliminate operator errors, which are the major contributor to sterilization process failures. Every perioperative registered nurse must recognize the importance of their role in improving patient safety by following policies and procedures and properly performing the steps of the sterilization process. They need to have the knowledge to understand what steps need to be performed and why. Up-to-date policies and procedures, training, competency testing, and ongoing education are essential to eliminating operator errors.

KNOW YOUR STEAM STERILIZER

Operator errors can also be eliminated by knowing what type of sterilizer cycles are available so you can choose the correct monitoring procedure and products and the correct cycle for the load contents. Two types of sterilizer cycles are available: gravity-displacement and dynamic-air-removal.

The gravity-displacement cycle is a "Type of sterilization cycle in which incoming steam displaces residual air through a port or drain in or near the bottom (usually) of the sterilizer chamber."[9] The dynamic-air-removal cycle is "One of two types of sterilization cycles in which air is removed from the chamber and the load by means of a series of pressure and vacuum excursions (prevacuum cycle) or by means of a series of steam flushes and pressure pulses above atmospheric pressure (steam-flush pressure-pulse [SFPP] cycle)."[10]

Sterilizers used today tend to have both types of cycles and several different time and temperature options for these cycles.

Knowing your steam sterilizer is also important because the ANSI/AAMI ST79 Section **10** on Quality Control discusses the recommendations for routine sterilizer efficacy monitoring (section 10.7) and sterilization qualification testing (section 10.8) according to the size and type of sterilizer used:

Sterilizers larger than 2 cubic feet (section 10.7.2, 10.8.2)
Table-top sterilizers (section 10.7.3, 10.8.3)
Flash sterilization cycles (section 10.7.4, 10.8.4).

It is important to further define flash sterilization. Flash sterilization is a "Process designed for the steam sterilization of patient care items for immediate use."[11] The flash sterilization process has expanded beyond its original intention of processing single, dropped instruments in an emergency situation. Originally, a dropped instrument was placed in an open surgical tray (eg, perforated, unwrapped instrument tray with no absorbent material) and processed for 3 minutes in a 270°F to 275°F (132°C–135°C) gravity steam sterilization cycle. Currently, flash sterilization is performed:

At 270°F–275°F (132°C–135°C)
In both gravity and dynamic-air-removal sterilizers (i.e., prevacuum or steam-flush pressure-pulse)
For 3 or more minutes
With no drying time
In many different types of packaging
    Perforated, mesh bottom, open, surgical tray
    Containment devices
        Protective organizing cases
        Rigid sterilization containers
    Single-wrapped surgical trays
By immediately transferring the processed items to the sterile field using aseptic technique.[12]

AORN is very clear in their *Recommended Practices for Sterilization in the Perioperative Practice Setting* that "Flash sterilization should not be used as a substitute for sufficient instrument inventory,"[13] and "Flash sterilization may be associated with increased risk of infection to patients because of pressure on personnel to eliminate one or more steps in the cleaning and sterilization process."[14] This example would be another source of operator error that leads to a sterilization process failure. In addition, AORN states that "Rigid sterilization containers designed and intended for flash-sterilization cycles should be used" to reduce the risk of contamination during transport and assist in presentation to the sterile field.[15]

Perioperative nurses must ensure they have the most up-to-date instructions for use of the sterilizer so that they know which cycles are available and the minimum time and temperature validated for each sterilizer cycle by the sterilizer manufacturer. They should obtain up-to-date instructions for use of all medical devices to ensure the sterilization cycle and dry time is appropriate for those devices. Some medical device manufacturers' may require a sterilization cycle that is longer than the cycle validated and recommended by the sterilizer manufacturer. These are called extended cycles, which are defined as "Steam sterilization cycle with longer exposure times, dry times, or both than those commonly provided by the sterilizer manufacturers (eg, whereas a normal cycle might be 4 minutes at 270°F, an extended cycle could be 15 minutes at 270°F)."[16]

Many manufacturers of complex medical devices do not provide any 270°F to 275°F (132°C–135°C) flash sterilization parameters because the cycle time is too long to be practical. Currently, too many operating rooms are not running a long enough cycle to produce products safe for patient use.

During a survey, perioperative nurses should be prepared for the Joint Commission surveyor to ask to see those up-to-date instructions for not only the sterilizer and the medical devices but also the packaging and monitoring products being used.[17] The Centers for Medicare and Medicaid Services (CMS) also will be asking to see these instructions. CMS released a memo to state survey directors on October 13, 2009, clarifying their position on flash sterilization for ambulatory surgery centers. "Routine flash sterilization in ambulatory surgery centers is acceptable, as long as the load is wrapped or contained and the facility follows manufacturers' instruction for all the devices involved."[18] Access the referenced Web sites for more information about Joint Commission and CMS surveys.

Perioperative registered nurses have the responsibility to follow all manufacturer's up-to-date instructions for use to ensure the correct sterilization cycle is used.

STERILIZATION PROCESS MONITORING DEVICES

Sterilization process monitoring devices include physical monitors, chemical indicators (CIs), and BIs.[19] Process challenge devices (PCDs; formally called *routine* or *challenge test packs*) are also used to assess the effectiveness of the sterilization process. A PCD is an "Item designed to constitute a defined resistance to a sterilization process and used to assess performance of the process."[20] A PCD could include:

A BI;
A BI and Class 5 integrating indicator (class of CI), or
A Class 5 integrating indicator.

All of these monitors are used to determine the effectiveness of the sterilization process, because they are in different locations in the sterilizer and load and they provide different types of information. For the processed items to be considered safe for patient use, all of the monitors should show the process was effective.

PHYSICAL MONITORING

Physical monitors include time, temperature, and pressure recorders such as chart displays, digital printouts, and gauge readings. Physical monitoring provides real-time confirmation that the sterilization conditions were achieved, a permanent record of those results, and the first indication of a failed sterilization process. For recording charts, the perioperative registered nurse who is running the sterilizer should ensure at the beginning of the cycle that the pen is functioning and mark the chart with the correct date and sterilizer number. For sterilizers with printouts, perioperative nurses should check to see that the printer is functioning and the cycle identification number is recorded.[21]

Too often in operating rooms people get busy and remove medical devices from the sterilizer when the cycle was never run. To ensure this does not happen, at the end of the cycle the perioperative registered nurse who opens the sterilizer should check the chart or printout to ensure the correct cycle was run for the load contents, that all the parameters are correct, and initial the chart.[21] If the correct cycle was not run and the parameters were not correct, the load should not be used.

Physical monitoring will not detect loading and packaging problems that can interfere with steam sterilization because these monitors only measure the chamber temperature at the drain and not the temperature inside each package. Therefore, a complete sterilization monitoring program includes not only physical monitors but also chemical and biological indicators.

CHEMICAL INDICATORS

CIs include the Bowie-Dick test and those used inside and outside each health care facility's assembled package or rigid container. **Table 1** includes the definition of each class of CI and the practical application. The class number has no hierarchical significance[22]; perioperative nurses are responsible for choosing the class of CI based on the information needed.

Bowie-Dick Testing

Perioperative nurses should check with the manufacturer of the sterilizer to see if the Bowie-Dick test (Class 2 CI) should be run. It does not need to be run in gravity-displacement or steam-flush pressure-pulse sterilizers. The Bowie-Dick test is run each day before the sterilizer is used in a 270°F to 275°F (132°C–135°C) prevacuum steam sterilizer to determine if air leaks, an inadequate vacuum, or noncondensable gases are present in the sterilizer (eg, air or gases from the boiler additives that enter the chamber with the steam and inhibit proper steam penetration).[23] This test also needs to be run daily when using a 270°F to 275°F (132°C–135°C) prevacuum steam sterilizer for flash sterilization.

Perioperative nurses should make sure to follow the manufacturer of the Bowie-Dick test pack and sterilizer instructions for use or the results will be invalid. The sterilizer cannot be placed into routine use unless the Bowie-Dick test sheet shows a pass. **Box 1** summarizes how the Bowie-Dick test pack should be run according to the ANSI/AAMI ST79 recommended practice.[24]

Perioperative registered nurses are responsible for following these instructions for running the Bowie-Dick tests so that the results are valid and the sterilizer can be placed into routine use for the day.

Internal Chemical Indicators

An internal CI (Class 3 single-variable, Class 4 multi-variable, or Class 5 integrating indicators) should be used inside each package, tray, or rigid sterilization container system to be sterilized in the area determined to be the least accessible to steam penetration.[25] The recommended practices state that Class 4 multi-variable and Class 5 integrating indicators provide more information than Class 3 single-variable indicators.[25]

The AORN *Recommended Practice for Sterilization in the Perioperative Practice Setting*, 2009 states "Class 5 chemical integrating indicators should be used within each sterilizer container or tray."[26] The AORN *Recommended Practices for Selection*

Table 1
Chemical indicator classes and practical application

Class	Definition	Practical Application
Class 1: Process Indicators	"intended for use with individual units, (eg, packs, containers) to indicate that the unit has been directly exposed to the sterilization process and to distinguish between processed and unprocessed units. These indicators are also referred to as external CIs."	Indicator tapes, indicator labels, and load cards are examples of external CI
Class 2: Indicators for Use in Specific Tests	"intended for use in specific test procedures (eg, the Bowie-Dick test) as defined in relevant sterilizer/ sterilization standards."	Bowie-Dick–type tests are specific tests used to evaluate the sterilizer performance
Class 3: Single-variable Indicators	"designed to react to one of the critical variables[a] and intended to indicate exposure to a sterilization process at a stated value of the chosen variable."	An example of a single-variable indicator is a temperature tube that contains a chemical pellet that melts at a specific temperature. Single-variable indicators may be used for pack control monitoring but would not provide as much information as a Class 4 or Class 5 CI. Single-variable indicators may also be used to determine that a specific temperature was reached at a specific location in the sterilizer chamber
Class 4: Multi-variable Indicators	"designed to react to two or more of the critical variables and intended to indicate exposure to a sterilization cycle at stated values[b] of the chosen variables."	Multi-variable indicators are used as internal CIs and are usually paper strips printed with a CI

| Class 5: Integrating Indicators | "designed to react to all critical variables, with the stated values having been generated to be equivalent to, or exceed, the performance requirements given in the ISO 11138 series for BIs." | Integrating indicators are the most precise of the internal CIs
Integrating indicators are used as internal CIs
They may also be used as an additional monitoring tool to release loads that do not contain implants
For this additional monitoring, the Class 5 integrating indicator must be used in the appropriate process challenge device should be used in the BI PCD for releasing implants |
| Class 6: Emulating Indicators | "cycle verification indicators designed to react to all critical variables of specified sterilization cycles, with the stated values having been generated from the critical variables of the specific sterilization process." | ANSI/AAMI ST79:2006, A1:2008, A2:2009 recommended practice "does not cover the use and application of Class 6 emulating indicators." |

Abbreviations: BI, biological indicator; CI, chemical indicator ink.

[a] Critical variables: "Parameters identified as being essential to the sterilization process (and requiring monitoring)." (definition 3.2)

[b] Stated value (SV): "'Value or values of a critical variable at which the indicator is designed to reach its endpoint as defined by the manufacturer.'" (definition 3.12) For example, a Class 5 Integrating Indicator with a stated value of 2.1 minutes at 135°C should reach its endpoint when tested at 135°C for 2.1 minutes in a resistometer."

Data from Definitions from the Association for the Advancement of Medical Instrumentation. Sterilization of health care products-chemical indicators-part 1: general requirements. ANSI/AAMI/ISO 11140-1:2005. Arlington (VA). Association for the Advancement of Medical Instrumentation. Comprehensive guide to steam sterilization and sterility assurance in health care facilities (Section 10.5.2.1). ANSI/AAMI ST79:2006, A1:2008 and A2:2009. Arlington (VA) 2006.

Box 1
Appropriate performance of the Bowie-Dick test

1. Run an empty cycle right before the Bowie-Dick test to preheat the sterilizer and purge air out of the lines, even if the sterilizer was never turned off.

2. Place one Bowie-Dick test pack horizontally in the front bottom section of the sterilizer rack near the door over the drain, but not on the floor or on top of a perforated tray. The sterilizer manufacturers recommend using the sterilizer rack at all times to prevent the formation of superheat, which could cause a failed Bowie-Dick test.

3. Run the test pack for 3.5 to 4 minutes at 270°F to 275°F (132°C–135°C), or the test sheet will be uniform even if the air pocket is present.

4. Read the physical monitors and initial the printout.

5. If the test sheet has a uniform color change, use the sterilizer.

6. If the test sheet does not have a uniform color change, retest the sterilizer.

7. If a second Bowie-Dick test is run and that sheet has a uniform color change, use the sterilizer.

8. If the second Bowie-Dick test does not have a uniform color change, do not use the sterilizer until the problem is identified.

9. The supervisor must determine if the sterilizer requires retesting or servicing, or can remain in use. The later section on Recall and Sterilizer Qualification Testing provides information on when and how to test the sterilizer before returning it to routine use.

---

and Use of Packaging Systems for Sterilization, 2009 suggests the following placement of internal CIs[27]:

> A CI in the geometric center not on the top of a wrapped pack or tray (**Fig. 1**)
> Two CIs inside rigid containers, one in each of two opposite corners of the inside basket (**Fig. 2**)
> Multilevel containers should have a CI placed in two opposite corners (eg, one in each of two corners) of each level (**Fig. 3**)
> A CI in center of each level of multilevel wrapped container sets (**Fig. 4**).

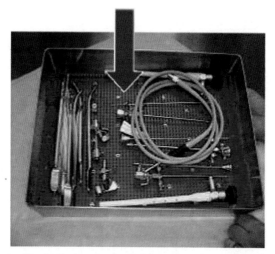

Fig. 1. Class 5 integrating indicators in geometric center not on top of wrapped tray.

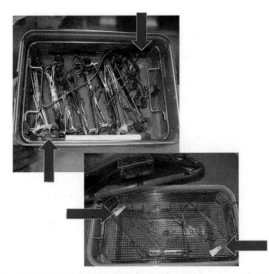

Fig. 2. Two Class 5 integrating indicators inside rigid containers, one in each of two opposite corners.

Because it is possible to have internal CIs change in some locations but not all in the same package or container, these items should be opened up on a back table to avoid contamination of the sterile field. The instruments should not be moved to the sterile field until it is determined that all the CIs have reached their end point response (eg, migration to pass or appropriate color).

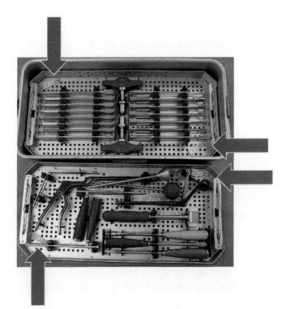

Fig. 3. Class 5 integrating indicator in two opposite corners on each level of a multilevel container set.

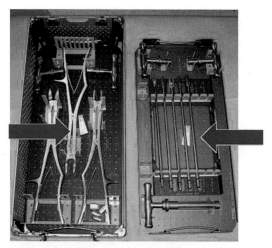

Fig. 4. Class 5 integrating indicator in center on each level of multilayer wrapped container sets.

Every perioperative registered nurse must be trained and their competency determined to ensure they know how to read the results of the internal CI. These nurses are the gatekeepers in the operating room, and are responsible for stopping the use of a package that suggests an inadequate steam sterilization process.

External Chemical Indicators

An external CI (Class 1) should be placed on the outside of each package unless the internal CI is visible (eg, peel pouches, open perforated surgical trays). "The purpose of an external CI is to differentiate between processed and unprocessed items, not to establish whether the parameters for adequate sterilization were met."[28]

After unloading the sterilizer, the external CI should be checked on each package. The tray, package, or container should not be released for use if the CI has not reached its end point response. The external CI should be checked again before the package or container is moved into the operating room suite.

BIOLOGICAL INDICATORS

"Biological indicators are the only sterilization process monitoring device that provides a direct measure of the lethality of the process."[29] CIs cannot replace the use of BIs because these sterilization monitoring devices do not contain spores and thus do not directly measure the lethality of a sterilization cycle.[30] BIs should be incubated according to the manufacturer's instructions and facility's policy and procedures.[29] Each day that a test BI is incubated, a control BI (not sterilized) from the same lot should be incubated in each auto-reader or incubator to "verify the presterilization viability of the test spores, the ability of the media to promote growth of the test spores, and the proper incubation temperature."[31] If the control BI is negative, the test results are invalid and should be repeated.

Perioperative registered nurses are responsible for ensuring that the test and control lot of the BI match and the manufacturer's instructions for incubation are followed.

FOUR LEVELS OF TESTING

ANSI/AAMI ST79 requires four levels of testing. Each level of testing is described below.

Routine Load Release for Nonimplant and Implant Loads

The placement of the BI PCD in the load will be the same as described for routine sterilizer efficacy monitoring.

Nonimplants

The following monitoring should be performed routinely for each load of nonimplants before it is released for use to ensure that the sterilization process was effective:

Physically monitor each load
Label every package with an external process indicator (Class 1)
Place an internal CI inside each package (Class 3, 4, or 5)
If desired, place a PCD in the chamber containing
   A BI
   A BI and a Class 5 integrating CI
   A Class 5 integrating CI
Evaluate all quality control measures and data at the conclusion of the sterilization
   cycle (this should be performed by an experienced, knowledgeable individual)
Release loads only if the criteria for release are present.[32]

Implants

The following monitoring should be performed routinely for each load of implants, which "should be quarantined until the results of the BI testing are available"[33]:

Physically monitor each load
Label every package with an external process indicator (Class 1)
Place an internal CI inside each package (Class 3, 4, or 5)
Monitor with a PCD containing a BI and a Class 5 integrating CI
Evaluate all quality control measures and data at the conclusion of the sterilization
   cycle (this should be performed by an experienced, knowledgeable individual)
Quarantine implant until BI is negative
Release loads only if the criteria for release are present.[34]

Premature release of implants before the BI result is available is "unacceptable and should be the exception, not the rule."[33] These should only be released when the health care facility's documented medical exceptions dictate.[33] Each medical exception should be documented using an implant exception form. ANSI/AAMI ST79 has an example of an exception form. The following information should be recorded for each implant that is prematurely released:

Name of:
   Implant prematurely released
   Patient
   Surgeon (some facilities have the surgeon sign this form)
Reason for premature release
What could have prevented premature release of the implant.[35]

All the sterilization process monitoring results for an implant should be documented and fully traceable to the patient on whom it is used or in whom it is implanted.[33,36]

"Flash sterilization of implants should not be used for implantable devices except in cases of emergency when no other option is available."[37] This process increases the risk of surgical site infections.[37] It is a major responsibility of a perioperative nurse to minimize patient risk for surgical site infections.[1] If implants continue to be released before BI results are available or implants continue to be flash sterilized, a risk analysis should be performed to determine how to eliminate these events to improve the outcome of the sterilization process and prevent surgical site infections.[38] Perioperative registered nurses should take the lead.

ROUTINE STERILIZER EFFICACY TESTING

Routine sterilizer efficacy monitoring is divided into sections based on the size and type of the sterilizer (larger than 2 cubic feet, table-top sterilizers, and flash sterilization cycles). Routine testing with a BI PCD "should be done at least weekly, but preferably every day that the sterilizer is in use" to ensure the steam sterilizer is effectively sterilizing medical devices.[39]

In addition each type of cycle for which a sterilizer is designed to be used must be routinely tested because each cycle creates a different challenge to air removal and steam penetration

Gravity-displacement at 132°C to 135°C (270°F–275°F)
Gravity-displacement at 121°C (250°F)
Dynamic-air-removal at 132°C to 135°C (270°F–275°F)
Flash at 132°C to 135°C (270°F–275°F)
Flash with single wrapper or other packaging.[30]

For example, if any of the above listed cycles are run routinely, a BI PCD should be run in each of those cycles weekly, preferably daily. The exception is "If a sterilizer will run the same type of cycle (eg, dynamic-air-removal at 132°C to 135°C [270°F to 275°F]) for different exposure times (eg, 4 minutes and 10 minutes), then only the shortest cycle time needs to be tested."[40] These different cycles to be tested may be found in sterilizers larger than 2 cubic feet, table-top sterilizers, and flash sterilization cycles.

For flash sterilization, each type of tray configuration routinely processed should be tested because each creates a different challenge to air removal and steam penetration during the sterilization process:

Perforated, mesh-bottom, open surgical tray
Rigid sterilization container system
Protective organizing case
Single-wrapped surgical tray.[41]

Therefore, if both an open surgical tray and a rigid sterilization container are routinely used, a BI should be tested at least weekly, but preferably every day that the sterilizer is used, in each of these types of packaging. A commercially available BI PCD is not available,[42] so the BI PCD should be prepared by the health care facility by placing a BI and one or more CIs inside each type of packaging used. See the AORN recommendations for placement of CIs discussed earlier as a guide for where to place BIs and CIs. These indicators should always be placed in the most challenging area of the packaging. The BI PCD is placed in an empty chamber on the bottom rack over the drain, which is the area that presents the greatest challenge because it minimizes the heat-up time and the lethality of the process.[43] A Bowie-Dick test should be run each morning if the flash sterilization cycle is a prevacuum running at 132°C to 135°C (270°F–275°F).

For sterilizers larger than 2 cubic feet, an AAMI 16 towel pack containing a BI and CI, or a commercially available disposable BI PCD cleared by the FDA for this intended use, should be run.[44] The BI PCD is placed in a full load on the bottom rack over the drain because this area presents the greatest challenge for the sterilization process that always includes the load.[45] Each type of cycle used should always be tested.[46]

For table-top sterilizers, commercial prepared BI PCDs are not available. A BI PCD should be prepared using the same type of package or tray routinely processed. "The package or tray considered to be the most difficult to sterilize should be selected from those most frequently processed" and should "contain the items normally present during routine sterilization"[47] For example, a BI PCD that includes multiple layers of dressing materials would be a greater challenge than an instrument in a peel pouch. The BI PCD should be placed in the center of the full load toward the front,[48] which is the coolest spot in the sterilizer and presents the greatest challenge.[48] The sterilizer manufacturer should be consulted for their placement recommendation. Each type of cycle used should be tested.[46]

Perioperative nurses are responsible for ensuring that all routine sterilizer efficacy testing is performed and performed correctly. To simplify these BI PCD monitoring requirements and reduce variability and the chance for operator errors, such as not testing all of the types of cycles and packaging used and every implant load, a BI PCD containing a Class 5 integrating indicator should be run in each load. This practice would be a universal standard of care.

STERILIZER QUALIFICATION TESTING

Sterilizer qualification testing is performed after an event has occurred, which could affect the performance of the sterilizer/utilities.[49] These events include:

Sterilizer installation
Sterilizer relocation
Sterilizer malfunctions
Sterilizer major repairs
    A major repair is a repair outside the scope of normal maintenance, including weld repairs of the pressure vessel, replacement of the chamber door or major piping assembly, or rebuilds or upgrades of controls. Normal preventive maintenance, such as the rebuilding of solenoid valves or the replacement of gaskets, is not considered major repair. Changes to the utilities connected to the sterilizer, such as those caused by a water main break, annual boiler maintenance, additional equipment loads, and installation of new boilers, should be treated as major repairs.
Sterilization process failures.[49]

Sterilizer qualification testing is performed in empty loads with the BI PCD over the drain for sterilizers greater than 2 cubic feet because that is the coldest spot and the greatest challenge.[50] For flash sterilizers, the BI PCD is placed over the drain in an empty sterilizer because that is the coolest spot in the chamber and it minimizes the heat-up time and the lethality of the process.[51] This testing is performed in a table-top sterilizer in full loads, which represents the greatest challenge because of the limited amount of water to create steam.[52]

For sterilizer qualification testing, a BI PCD is run in three consecutive cycles, one right after the other, followed by a BD test that is run in three consecutive empty cycles one right after the other, if the sterilizer is a prevacuum.[49] The sterilizer should not be placed into use until all of the monitoring results indicate an effective sterilization process. Perioperative registered nurses are responsible for ensuring that this sterilizer qualification testing is performed when these events occur, and performed correctly so the efficacy of the sterilizer is verified before it is put into routine use.

PRODUCT TESTING (PERIODIC PRODUCT QUALITY ASSURANCE TESTING OF ROUTINELY PROCESSED ITEMS)

Product testing is performed to ensure the effectiveness of the sterilization process and avoid wet packs. Product testing should be performed on an ongoing basis and periodically to test routinely sterilized products.[53] "Before newly purchased or loaner sets are placed into routine use, they should be evaluated to determine if the existing product testing is applicable to these sets."[53] In addition, "product testing should always be performed when major changes are made in packaging, wraps, or load configuration, such as dimensional changes, weight changes, or changes in the type or material of packaging or wrapper."[53] Product testing should be performed because:

> *"The standardized PCD (BI challenge pack) of 10.7.2.1 presents a known challenge to the sterilization process. However, this pack does not necessarily reflect the same challenge as the items routinely processed in a health care facility. Therefore, product testing is recommended as part of a complete quality assurance program to ensure the effectiveness of the sterilization process and to avoid wet packs."[53]*

This testing should be performed by the sterile processing department staff. Perioperative nurses are responsible for helping to

Provide up-to-date package inserts for all newly purchased or loaner sets
Arrange product testing for those sets before they are placed into routine use
Ensure product testing is performed on any of the major changes listed above before those changes are placed into routine use.

RECALL

The objective of a recall is to "expedite the retrieval of processed items that are suspected to be nonsterile and to ensure adequate follow-up actions such as quarantine of the sterilizer, notification of physicians and affected clinical departments, and surveillance of patients."[54] Each health care facility should have written policies and procedures for the recall of items from issued or stored sterilization processes.[54] These policies and procedures "should be developed for compliance with the Safe Medical Device Act of 1990 as it pertains to failures of reusable medical devices (i.e., the Medical Device Reporting [MDR] regulations of 21 CFR 803)."[54]

When to recall will depend on the root cause of the sterilization process failure. The second set of amendments (A2:2009) published for ANSI/AAMI ST79 in August 2009 included additional information to assist in development of a recall policy and procedure.[55] A decision tree for conducting investigations of steam sterilization process failures (Fig. 12) and a troubleshooting checklist for identifying reasons for steam sterilization process failures (Table 8) were added.[56] This checklist includes operator errors and sterilizer or utility malfunctions.

The decision tree shows how to respond to failed physical monitors and CIs in addition to BIs and what additional testing is required. A recall back to the last negative BI should be initiated if the failure is not immediately identified. The action steps now state:

"(b) If the cause of failure is immediately identified (usually operator error) and confined to one load or one item in the load (ie, an item with a nonresponsive internal CI), the cause of the failure should be corrected and the load should be reprocessed. If the cause of the failure is not immediately identified, the load should be quarantined, and all loads back to the last negative BI should be recalled. Items in these loads should be retrieved, if possible, and reprocessed.... The sterilizer in question should be taken out of service for further investigation of root causes."[56]

"(d) The heads of the microbiology department, sterilizing department, and infection prevention and control department, or their designees, with appropriate facility maintenance and sterilizer service personnel, should attempt to determine the root cause of the sterilization process failure and arrange for corrective action."[57]

The decision tree provided in section 10.7.5.1 of the ANSI/AAMI ST79 *Comprehensive Guide to Steam Sterilization and Sterility Assurance in Health Care Facilities* states what testing is needed to place the sterilizer back into routine use depending on the root cause of the failure:

Can be attributed to a cause other than a sterilizer/utilities malfunction: correct the error and return the sterilizer to service

Cannot be attributed to a cause other than a sterilizer/utilities malfunction and the repair is minor: the sterilizer can be returned to service without conducting qualification testing

Can be attributed to a sterilizer/utilities malfunction that requires a major repair: sterilizer qualification testing should be performed before the sterilizer is replaced into routine use (see the earlier section on Sterilizer Qualification Testing).[57]

A recall order includes the following information:

A list of all items processed back to the last negative BI

Lot numbers of items to be recalled

Identification of persons or departments to whom the order is addressed

Information required to be recorded in terms of kind and quantity of products recalled

Specify action to be taken by the persons receiving the order, such as returning or destroying products.[58]

Perioperative registered nurses are responsible for following the recall order, because retrieval of these items is an important step in preventing surgical site infections.

DOCUMENTATION

Documentation establishes accountability. It can be performed using a paper or digitized system. "Digitization of this process will allow quick access to load information, facilitating a quick response."[59] Perioperative nurses are responsible for documenting any events they were involved with, including:

Each product processed for identification and traceability

Monitoring results of each load

Early release of implants

Results of sterilizer qualification testing after installation and maintenance of sterilizer/utilities

Results of product testing

Recall results

Medical device manufacturer's instructions for use

SUMMARY

The goal of a perioperative registered nurse is to minimize patient risk for surgical site infection. This goal can be achieved by keeping up-to-date on the recommended procedures that establish the clinical practice for improving the outcome of the steam sterilization process. This improvement involves development and adherence to policies and procedures, training, competency testing, and ongoing education to eliminate operator errors, which are the primary reason for a sterilization process failure. Perioperative registered nurses must understand why and how the steam sterilization process should be monitored so that medical devices not properly sterilized do not contact the patient. They are the gatekeepers.

REFERENCES

1. Association of periOperative Registered Nurses. Recommended practices for sterilization in perioperative practice settings [purpose]. AORN Perioperative Standards and Recommended Practices. Denver (CO): 2009.
2. Association for Professionals in Infection Control and Epidemiology. Available at: http://www.apic.org/Content/NavigationMenu/PracticeGuidance/TargetingZero/ Targeting_Zero2.htm. Accessed June 8, 2010.
3. Centers for Disease Control. Guideline for Prevention of Surgical Site Infection. Atlanta (GA): 1999. p. 261.
4. Association for the Advancement of Medical Instrumentation. Comprehensive guide to steam sterilization and sterility assurance in health care facilities ANSI/ AAMI ST79:2006, A1:2008 and A2:2009. Arlington (VA): Section 11.3.2.
5. Association for the Advancement of Medical Instrumentation. Comprehensive guide to steam sterilization and sterility assurance in health care facilities ANSI/ AAMI ST79:2006, A1:2008 and A2:2009. Arlington (VA): Section 11.2.3.
6. Association of periOperative Registered Nurses. Recommended Practices for Sterilization in Perioperative Practice Settings [policy template]. AORN Perioperative Standards and Recommended Practices. Denver (CO): 2009.
7. The Joint Commission. Hospital Accreditation Standard. Chicago (IL): 2009. p. 127, 114, 118, 237.
8. Association for the Advancement of Medical Instrumentation. Comprehensive guide to steam sterilization and sterility assurance in health care facilities ANSI/ AAMI ST79:2006, A1:2008 and A2:2009. Arlington (VA): Section 4.3.1.
9. Association for the Advancement of Medical Instrumentation. Comprehensive guide to steam sterilization and sterility assurance in health care facilities ANSI/ AAMI ST79:2006, A1:2008 and A2:2009. Arlington (VA): Definition 2.27.
10. Association for the Advancement of Medical Instrumentation. Comprehensive guide to steam sterilization and sterility assurance in health care facilities ANSI/ AAMI ST79:2006, A1:2008 and A2:2009. Arlington (VA): Definition 2.26.
11. Association for the Advancement of Medical Instrumentation. Comprehensive guide to steam sterilization and sterility assurance in health care facilities ANSI/ AAMI ST79:2006, A1:2008 and A2:2009. Arlington (VA): Definition 2.50.

12. Association for the Advancement of Medical Instrumentation. Comprehensive guide to steam sterilization and sterility assurance in health care facilities ANSI/ AAMI ST79:2006, A1:2008 and A2:2009. Arlington (VA): Introduction/Overview, Section 8.6.2.

13. Association of periOperative Registered Nurses. Recommended Practices for Sterilization in Perioperative Practice Settings. AORN Perioperative Standards and Recommended Practices. Denver (CO); 2009: Recommendation IV.a.

14. Association of periOperative Registered Nurses. Recommended Practices for Sterilization in Perioperative Practice Settings. AORN Perioperative Standards and Recommended Practices. Denver (CO); 2009: Recommendation IV.

15. Association of periOperative Registered Nurses. Recommended Practices for Sterilization in Perioperative Practice Settings. AORN Perioperative Standards and Recommended Practices. Denver (CO); 2009: Recommendation IV.e.

16. Association for the Advancement of Medical Instrumentation. Process challenge devices/test packs for use in health care facilities AAMI TIR31:2008. Arlington (VA): Definition 3.7.

17. The Joint Commission. Update on The Joint Commission's Position on Steam Sterilization. Available at: http://search.jointcommission.org/search?q= Flash%20sterilization&site=All-Sites&client=jcaho_frontend&output=xml_no_ dtd&proxystylesheet=jcaho_frontend. Accessed April 26, 2010.

18. Outpatient Surgery E-Weekly. CMS OKs Routine Flashing for Wrapped Loads. Available at: http://www.outpatientsurgery.net/newsletter/eweekly/2009/10/13. Accessed April 26, 2010.

19. Association for the Advancement of Medical Instrumentation. Comprehensive guide to steam sterilization and sterility assurance in health care facilities ANSI/AAMI ST79:2006, A1:2008 and A2:2009. Arlington (VA): Section 10.4, Table 7.

20. Association for the Advancement of Medical Instrumentation. Comprehensive guide to steam sterilization and sterility assurance in health care facilities ANSI/ AAMI ST79:2006, A1:2008 and A2:2009. Arlington (VA): Definition 2.100.

21. Association for the Advancement of Medical Instrumentation. Comprehensive guide to steam sterilization and sterility assurance in health care facilities ANSI/ AAMI ST79:2006, A1:2008 and A2:2009. Arlington (VA): Section 10.5.1.

22. Association for the Advancement of Medical Instrumentation. Sterilization of health care products-Chemical indicators-Part 1: General requirements ANSI/ AAMI/ISO 11140–1:2005. Arlington (VA): 3.

23. Association for the Advancement of Medical Instrumentation. Comprehensive guide to steam sterilization and sterility assurance in health care facilities ANSI/ AAMI ST79:2006, A1:2008 and A2:2009. Arlington (VA): Section 10.7.6.1.

24. Association for the Advancement of Medical Instrumentation. Comprehensive guide to steam sterilization and sterility assurance in health care facilities ANSI/ AAMI ST79:2006, A1:2008 and A2:2009. Arlington (VA): Section 10.7.6.

25. Association for the Advancement of Medical Instrumentation. Comprehensive guide to steam sterilization and sterility assurance in health care facilities ANSI/ AAMI ST79:2006, A1:2008 and A2:2009. Arlington (VA): Section 10.5.2.2.2.

26. Association of periOperative Registered Nurses. Recommended Practices for Sterilization in Perioperative Practice Settings. AORN Perioperative Standards and Recommended Practices. Denver (CO); 2009: Recommendation IV.c.3.

27. Association of periOperative Registered Nurses. Recommended Practices for Sterilization in Perioperative Practice Settings. AORN Perioperative Standards and Recommended Practices. Denver (CO); 2009: Recommendation IX.

28. Association for the Advancement of Medical Instrumentation. Comprehensive guide to steam sterilization and sterility assurance in health care facilities ANSI/ AAMI ST79:2006, A1:2008 and A2:2009. Arlington (VA): Section 10.5.2.2.1.

29. Association for the Advancement of Medical Instrumentation. Comprehensive guide to steam sterilization and sterility assurance in health care facilities ANSI/ AAMI ST79:2006, A1:2008 and A2:2009. Arlington (VA): Section 10.5.3.1.

30. Association for the Advancement of Medical Instrumentation. Comprehensive guide to steam sterilization and sterility assurance in health care facilities ANSI/ AAMI ST79:2006, A1:2008 and A2:2009. Arlington (VA): Section 10.5.3.2.

31. Association for the Advancement of Medical Instrumentation. Comprehensive guide to steam sterilization and sterility assurance in health care facilities ANSI/ AAMI ST79:2006, A1:2008 and A2:2009. Arlington (VA): Section 10.7.2.3, 10.7.3.3, 10.7.4.3, 10.8.2.3, 10.8.3.3, 10.8.4.3.

32. Association for the Advancement of Medical Instrumentation. Comprehensive guide to steam sterilization and sterility assurance in health care facilities ANSI/ AAMI ST79:2006, A1:2008 and A2:2009. Arlington (VA): Section 10.5.4, 10.6.2.

33. Association for the Advancement of Medical Instrumentation. Comprehensive guide to steam sterilization and sterility assurance in health care facilities ANSI/ AAMI ST79:2006, A1:2008 and A2:2009. Arlington (VA): Section 10.6.3.

34. Association for the Advancement of Medical Instrumentation. Comprehensive guide to steam sterilization and sterility assurance in health care facilities ANSI/ AAMI ST79:2006, A1:2008 and A2:2009. Arlington (VA): Section 10.5.4, 10.6.3.

35. Association for the Advancement of Medical Instrumentation. Comprehensive guide to steam sterilization and sterility assurance in health care facilities ANSI/ AAMI ST79:2006, A1:2008 and A2:2009. Arlington (VA): Annex L.

36. Association of periOperative Registered Nurses. Recommended Practices for Sterilization in Perioperative Practice Settings. AORN Perioperative Standards and Recommended Practices. Denver (CO); 2009: Recommendation Practice IV.i.

37. Association of periOperative Registered Nurses. Recommended Practices for Sterilization in Perioperative Practice Settings. AORN Perioperative Standards and Recommended Practices. Denver (CO); 2009: Recommendation Practice IV.h.1.

38. Association for the Advancement of Medical Instrumentation. Comprehensive guide to steam sterilization and sterility assurance in health care facilities ANSI/ AAMI ST79:2006, A1:2008 and A2:2009. Arlington (VA): Section 11.2.2.

39. Association for the Advancement of Medical Instrumentation. Comprehensive guide to steam sterilization and sterility assurance in health care facilities ANSI/ AAMI ST79:2006, A1:2008 and A2:2009. Arlington (VA): Section 10.5.2.

40. Association for the Advancement of Medical Instrumentation. Comprehensive guide to steam sterilization and sterility assurance in health care facilities ANSI/ AAMI ST79:2006, A1:2008 and A2:2009. Arlington (VA): Section 10.5.3.2, 10.7.4.1.

41. Association for the Advancement of Medical Instrumentation. Comprehensive guide to steam sterilization and sterility assurance in health care facilities ANSI/ AAMI ST79:2006, A1:2008 and A2:2009. Arlington (VA): Section 10.7.4.1.

42. Association for the Advancement of Medical Instrumentation. Comprehensive guide to steam sterilization and sterility assurance in health care facilities ANSI/ AAMI ST79:2006, A1:2008 and A2:2009. Arlington (VA): Section 10.5.4.

43. Association for the Advancement of Medical Instrumentation. Comprehensive guide to steam sterilization and sterility assurance in health care facilities ANSI/ AAMI ST79:2006, A1:2008 and A2:2009. Arlington (VA): Section 10.7.4.2.

44. Association for the Advancement of Medical Instrumentation. Comprehensive guide to steam sterilization and sterility assurance in health care facilities ANSI/ AAMI ST79:2006, A1:2008 and A2:2009. Arlington (VA): Section 10.7.2.

45. Association for the Advancement of Medical Instrumentation. Comprehensive guide to steam sterilization and sterility assurance in health care facilities ANSI/ AAMI ST79:2006, A1:2008 and A2:2009. Arlington (VA): Section 10.7.2.2.

46. Association for the Advancement of Medical Instrumentation. Comprehensive guide to steam sterilization and sterility assurance in health care facilities ANSI/ AAMI ST79:2006, A1:2008 and A2:2009. Arlington (VA): Section 10.7.1.

47. Association for the Advancement of Medical Instrumentation. Comprehensive guide to steam sterilization and sterility assurance in health care facilities ANSI/ AAMI ST79:2006, A1:2008 and A2:2009. Arlington (VA): Section 10.7.3.

48. Association for the Advancement of Medical Instrumentation. Comprehensive guide to steam sterilization and sterility assurance in health care facilities ANSI/ AAMI ST79:2006, A1:2008 and A2:2009. Arlington (VA): Section 10.7.3.2.

49. Association for the Advancement of Medical Instrumentation. Comprehensive guide to steam sterilization and sterility assurance in health care facilities ANSI/ AAMI ST79:2006, A1:2008 and A2:2009.Arlington (VA): Section 10.8.1.

50. Association for the Advancement of Medical Instrumentation. Comprehensive guide to steam sterilization and sterility assurance in health care facilities ANSI/ AAMI ST79:2006, A1:2008 and A2:2009. Arlington (VA): Section 10.8.2.2.

51. Association for the Advancement of Medical Instrumentation. Comprehensive guide to steam sterilization and sterility assurance in health care facilities ANSI/ AAMI ST79:2006, A1:2008 and A2:2009. Arlington (VA): Section 10.8.4.2.

52. Association for the Advancement of Medical Instrumentation. Comprehensive guide to steam sterilization and sterility assurance in health care facilities ANSI/ AAMI ST79:2006, A1:2008 and A2:2009. Arlington (VA): Section 10.8.3.2.

53. Association for the Advancement of Medical Instrumentation. Comprehensive guide to steam sterilization and sterility assurance in health care facilities ANSI/ AAMI ST79:2006, A1:2008 and A2:2009. Arlington (VA): Section 10.9.

54. Association for the Advancement of Medical Instrumentation. Comprehensive guide to steam sterilization and sterility assurance in health care facilities ANSI/ AAMI ST79:2006, A1:2008 and A2:2009. Arlington (VA): Section 10.11.1.

55. Association for the Advancement of Medical Instrumentation. Comprehensive guide to steam sterilization and sterility assurance in health care facilities ANSI/ AAMI ST79:2006, A1:2008 and A2:2009. Arlington (VA): Section 10.7.5.

56. Association for the Advancement of Medical Instrumentation. Comprehensive guide to steam sterilization and sterility assurance in health care facilities ANSI/ AAMI ST79:2006, A1:2008 and A2:2009. Arlington (VA): Section 10.7.5.1, Figure 12, Table 8.

57. Association for the Advancement of Medical Instrumentation. Comprehensive guide to steam sterilization and sterility assurance in health care facilities ANSI/AAMI ST79:2006, A1:2008 and A2:2009. Arlington (VA): Section 10.7.5.1, Figure 12.

58. Association for the Advancement of Medical Instrumentation. Comprehensive guide to steam sterilization and sterility assurance in health care facilities ANSI/ AAMI ST79:2006, A1:2008 and A2:2009. Arlington (VA): Section 10.11.3.

59. Association for the Advancement of Medical Instrumentation. Comprehensive guide to steam sterilization and sterility assurance in health care facilities ANSI/ AAMI ST79:2006, A1:2008 and A2:2009. Arlington (VA): Section 10.3.2.

Regulations that Impact Disinfection and Sterilization Processes

ALPHA Patrol: Keeping Health Care Safe for Everyone

Carla McDermott, RN, BS, CNOR, CRCST

KEYWORDS

• Disinfection • Sterilization • Regulatory agencies

"Time out" no longer means a corner for placement of errant children. Communication, continuous quality improvement, safer patient care, and integration of services are a day-to-day reality. Every clinical service depends, at some point while providing patient care, on the Sterile Processing and Materiel Management (SP/MM) department. All reusable instruments, mobile equipment, and disposable supplies are facilitated in some way by SP/MM. They enable clinicians to provide the highest quality care. They are a vital link in bringing health to patients.[1]

The operating room (OR) suite historically was a "closed environment." Other than employees and patients, not many ventured beyond the OR's double doors. Through the 1980s, surveyors from the Joint Commission on Accreditation of Hospitals (JCAH) met with upper management and department heads in conference rooms. They talked at length and reviewed committee meeting minutes and records.[2] Over time, this reality has changed. Evolution and education of the public have increased the scrutiny of the activities performed inside the OR.

Today the Joint Commission, as they have been known since 2007,[2] uses a more physical and widespread survey process. Surveyors actually walk about the facility, question workers to validate education and ongoing quality improvement participation, and interview patients to validate their participation in improving their quality of life through health care. The Tracer Methodology[3] of survey and institution of

Baycare Healthcare System, South Florida Baptist Hospital, 601 North Alexander Street, Plant City, FL 33565, USA
E-mail address: carla.mcdermott@baycare.org

Perioperative Nursing Clinics 5 (2010) 347–353
doi:10.1016/j.cpen.2010.04.002
1556-7931/10/$ – see front matter © 2010 Elsevier Inc. All rights reserved.

periopnursing.theclinics.com

unannounced surveys has bought the surveyors directly into the operating rooms and other procedures locations. Direct observation and personal contact with everyone involved in patient care is the new experience.

APLHA PATROLS WHO KEEP A GUARDIAN EYE ON THE PRACTICES OF DISINFECTION AND STERILIZATION

Functions of the SP/MM department are regulated and monitored by a variety of over-seers beyond the Joint Commission. Although participation in JC accreditation is technically voluntary, facilities who desire payment for providing services to Medicare and Medicaid clients must first be JC accredited.[4] Other agencies, referred to in this article as the ALPHA Patrol, providing oversight and having established mandatory regulations include the Occupational Safety and Health Administration (OSHA), Centers for Medicare and Medicaid Services (CMS), Centers for Disease Control and Prevention (CDC), Environmental Protection Agency (EPA), Food and Drug Administration (FDA), and Agency for Healthcare Administration (AHCA).

OSHA, established in 1970 by the US Department of Labor, works to ensure safe work places for all employees.[5] The statutes established are law, therefore mandatory. Noncompliance with these statutes can cause severe fines to be levied against the facility and endanger JC accreditation. They are well recognized in health care facili-ties for the Bloodborne Pathogens Standard established in 1991 and Needlestick Safety and Prevention Act in 2001.[6] The statute regulating the use and monitoring of ethylene oxide (ETO) for sterilization is known as Title 29 of the Code of Federal Regulations (CFR) Part 1910. 1047.[7]

The US Department of Health and Human Services (HHS) was established in 1980. The mission is to protect the health of all Americans and provide essential human services.[8] The department includes more than 300 programs, with several agencies that impact hospitals. These include CMS, FDA, and CDC.[8]

In 1970, the EPA was established by the US government.[9] Their impact on SP/MM includes the chemicals used to clean, disinfect, and sterilize products as well as the product's disposal stream. The chemicals are hazardous to the environment if used or disposed of incorrectly. Strict adherence to the labeled practices of use and disposal are required. In some instances, even the shipping containers must be rendered harmless before disposal.[10] Many hospitals elected to discontinue use of facility-operated incinerators, further complicating the waste disposal stream and increased expense. Maintaining a central file of the Material Safety Data Sheet and manufacturer's instruction for storage, use, and disposal of all products helps ensure education and compliance of staff. A master file may be established and maintained with the facility's designated safety division; however, a central department file is most helpful when staff can access it easily in the event of an exposure or spill.

The FDA, established in 1906, regulates among other items, medical products. It is illegal to alter a medical device. This includes the device being sterilized and the ster-ilization device.[11] Reuse of devices labeled for "single use only" is also regulated by the FDA.[12]

Another federal entity active in SP/MM is AHCA. All health care facilities are required to be licensed by the government. Although AHCA's primary function is inspection of new and renovated facility constructions, annual facility inspections are also per-formed. This annual Life Safety Inspection works with OSHA to help ensure that facil-ities continue to be safe for workers and patients.[13] For example, if your facility elected to install a new ETO sterilizer, permits, inspections, and/or testing would be required by 4 agencies: AHCA, OSHA, EPA, and FDA.

WHAT IS ALPHA PATROL LOOKING FOR?

When one of these agencies comes into your facility they are looking for quality, regulatory compliance, standards compliance, validation of your operation, and evidence of self-monitoring. Signs of quality include having operating parameters and services well defined. Another sign of quality is having the mission and goals of the department listed. These 2 items will also provide direction for the entire team. The surveyors/inspectors will be looking to see that the department is clean, neat, and in good physical repair. It is as if they equate care of the employees and department as a reflection of the quality of patient care that is provided.

Record keeping is paramount for regulatory and standards compliance. Records need to demonstrate consistent adherence to all relevant statutes and departmental policies. For example, provision of ETO sterilization requires extensive use records, employee education, service area leak testing, employee exposure monitoring, and health screening. These records must be maintained for 30 years beyond termination of employee service.[7] Such stringent regulation and requirements are part of the reason many facilities are moving away from providing ETO sterilization. Failure to adequately research the facilities need for ETO service and appropriateness of other available alternative sterilization methods has led them to resume use of ETO or outsource this service. Other sterilization methods do not require such complex monitoring. Depending on your state and facility requirements, records of other sterilization processes may need to be retained for only 3, 5, or 7 years.

OSHA designates through the Hazard Communication Plan that all employees who have contact with, or work in the vicinity of ETO, peracetic acid, gluteraldehyde, and hydrogen peroxide gas plasma products also receive annual review of the hazards and safety procedures associated with each product.[4,5] Incorporating this with the annual performance appraisal or review can streamline some of the documentation.

One point of standards compliance that will be in the forefront of surveyors/inspectors' vision is documentation of education and proficiency. Bay Pines Veterans Hospital had problems that stemmed from not complying with manufacturers' instructions and not providing appropriate training regarding cleaning and sterilization of flexible fiberoptic endoscopes (FFE) scopes. The Department of Veterans Affairs (VA), Office of Inspector General, report released in June 2009 indicated a huge gap in compliance with the manufacturer's instructions for cleaning, disinfecting, and sterilizing of FFE. Less than 50% of the VA's endoscopy technicians had documented training/competency to perform these functions. This lack of effective training lead to substandard disinfecting and sterilizing of the FFEs. This recently affected approximately 10,000 military veterans.[14] These patients, in several VA facilities, have potentially been exposed to a number of communicable bloodborne pathogens. An August 2009 article in the *Army Times* indicated status changes of the patients who were subsequently tested. To date, 8 people with HIV, 12 people with Hepatitis B, and 37 people with Hepatitis C await proof their infections were directly caused by these errors in processing.[15] Appropriate education must be provided for each type of equipment processed. A documented return demonstration of successfully completing the processing steps validates the proficiency. Documentation of new hire orientation; education for new products, devices, and processes; and mandatory annual review can keep a manager very busy.[16]

Agencies that inspect or survey health care facilities will also be looking for evidence of validation. They are looking for "measures of success" related to operation and services.[17] Straightforward validation of sterilization cycles is common. Load contents, cycles, and parameters are everyday records of validation.

Biologic/chemical monitoring of select cycles validates correct operation of the equipment in use. It is also important to validate the recall procedure associated with each specific sterilization process. Using an actual event or staging an event will provide validation that the process is functional and adequate. Failures identified here provide opportunities to improve service. Other processes that require validation include any major renovation or repair of sterilization equipment. Changing packaging systems or products, such as rigid containers or wrapping materials, should also be validated as effective with use of your facilities equipment. Changing products for cleaning, disinfection, or lubrication should also be validated. Even if your facility does not experience frequent changes of this type, periodic documented monitoring of these processes will assure surveyors/inspectors of your level of commitment to high-quality care.

WHAT IMPACT CAN ALPHA PATROLS HAVE ON YOUR FACILITY?

Each of these agencies has one goal foremost on their priority list: provision of safe, appropriate, high-quality care. They arrive in our facilities at different times, by different means, for many different reasons. Their goal is always the same as our own, to ensure quality care is provided. The ultimate impact of every survey and inspection is an improvement in patient care.[17]

When things go awry, and they will occasionally, federal and state agencies have the authority to levy fines for infractions of the statutes/standards. The dollar amount of the fine is determined by severity of the infraction, number of like infractions found at the time, and their level of concern for potential harm to workers or patients.[18]

CMS can reduce the amount of funding the facility receives for services rendered to Medicare and Medicaid patients. Adhering to published CMS standards of quality care maintains the level of funding. A reduction reflects an inability to meet minimal expectations of care. For example, patients who are undergoing joint replacement surgery are expected to receive an appropriate intravenous antibiotic within the hour before incision. When this expectation is not met consistently, CMS funding can be reduced.[19] The goal here is delivery of appropriate, high-quality care that is evidence based. No one wants less for their patients, or to be paid less for their efforts.

Extreme consequences, including immediate closure of a facility or service is possible. Action of this magnitude reflects eminent life-threatening circumstances for the patients or staff. It is a rare, but not unheard of occurrence that can be levied by state or federal agencies.[20]

Focusing on the primary goal of providing safe, high-quality care will minimize trepidation when interacting with members of the ALPHA Patrol. They exist to protect all health care recipients and providers.

WHAT RESOURCES EXIST TO HELP MEET ALPHA PATROL'S DISINFECTION AND STERILIZATION STANDARDS?

Providing disinfection and sterilization services in a health care setting is a noble undertaking that seldom receives the recognition it deserves.[2] Regulations, statutes, standards, and recommendations for practice are abundant, seemingly never ending. They do not come packaged in a neat little box or computer file folder. Resources do exist to streamline your quest for excellence and dealing with the APLHA Patrols.

The first resource available is directly from the equipment or product manufacturer. Initial training before placement into use is generally provided by the manufacturer. One caveat here is to ensure the education is provided by a capable clinical educator, rather than the sales representative. The educational materials should also be available in print or audiovisual format for use in subsequent orientation and annual update programs.

OSHA offers educational products that are helpful when included in primary training for employees new to the disinfection and sterilization environment, as well as annual education update programs. These are available through the OSHA Web site (www.osha.gov).

The Association of Perioperative Registered Nurses (AORN) published the Perioperative Standards and Recommended Practices, 2009 edition,[21] that touch many points of interest. The publication contains 6 documents specifically addressing disinfection and sterilization recommended practices. Membership in AORN also provides access to subject matter experts, researchers, and other professional support. In particular, the Specialty Assembly for Sterile Processing/Materials Management was established to provide a networking forum for communication and specialized education programs. It serves as a meeting ground for perioperative managers, nurses, and SP/MM personnel. Contact them at www.aorn.org.

One comprehensive source for disinfection and sterilization standards is commonly known as ST79, published by the Association for the Advancement of Medical Instrumentation (AAMI) in league with the American National Standards Institute (ANSI).[22] It is a combination of several previously singular documents of AAMI officially titled "Comprehensive Guide to Steam Sterilization and Sterility Assurance in Healthcare Facilities ANSI/AAMI ST79:2006." For managers new to disinfection and sterilization services, this is a wellspring introduction. For those with more experience, it may be where they discover the roots of their labor and rationale for their efforts. The Web address is www.aami.org.

The International Association of Healthcare Central Service and Materiels Management (IAHCSMM) offers training materials prepared for several levels of participants.[23] A facility manager who does not have a primary educator for surgical services or SP will find turnkey products to assist with preparing employees to perform the vital functions of disinfection and sterilization. ST79 recommends that anyone who operates a sterilization system (steam, peracetic acid, gas plasma), regardless of their practice setting, receive education specific to the equipment and documented competency. Through IAHCSMM is access to the following publications: Central Service Technical Manual, Instructor's Guide for the Central Service Technical Manual, Supervision Principles Manual, Instrument Specialist Guide & Workbook, Facilitator's Guide for Instrument Specialist Guide, CS Orientation Guide, and Exx Cel Plus education modules. The Web address is www.iahcsmm.org. Access to Central Service (CS) education is also available through a partnership of IAHCSMM with Purdue University in an online format or traditional correspondence course format (www.continuinged.purdue.edu/media/cssp/). Membership offers access to subject matter experts, experienced CS educators, international and local chapter support, education, and the opportunity to share knowledge.[23]

Everyone who works in disinfection and sterilization is truly an infection prevention practitioner. The Association of Professionals in Infection Control (APIC) was established in 1972. The organization is committed to "improving patient care, preventing adverse outcomes, and minimizing occupational hazards associated with the delivery of health care."[24] Membership in APIC provides network support of more than 10,000 members. APIC offers several educational courses and products available through www.apic.org.

SUMMARY

Providing disinfection and sterilization services can be a monumental task. This is especially true for the novice who is just beginning this professional journey. It is a vital link in the efforts to provide safe health care. The medical community has been trying since ancient times to cure illness and improve the health of all people. Research and experience has taught many lessons along the way. The standards and recommended practices of these various agencies are a reflection of the lessons learned. They help guide everyday efforts toward a collective goal of safe, evidence-based, and high-quality health care, a quest perfectly aligned with AORN's own mission statement for patient safety.[24]

REFERENCES

1. CS' vital role in patient safety driven home at fall meeting. Healthcare Purchasing News Jan 2005. Available at: http://findarticles.com/p/articles/mi_mOBPC/is_1_29/ai_n8708452/. Accessed September 1, 2009.
2. A journey through the history of the Joint Commission. The Joint Commission web site. Available at: http://www.jointcommission.org/AboutUs/joint_commission_history.htm. updated August 25, 2009. Accessed September 1, 2009.
3. The Joint Commission. Available at: http://www.jointcommission.org/AboutUs/Fact_Sheets/Tracer_Methodology.htm. Accessed March 6, 2010.
4. Franko F. The importance of the Joint Commission – Health policy issues – Joint Commission Accreditation of Healthcare Organizations. AORN J 2002. Available at: http://findarticles.com/p/articles/mi_mOFSL/is_6_75/ai_88576001/. Accessed September 1, 2009.
5. Introduction to OSHA. Princeton University web site. Available at: http://web.princeton.edu/sites/ehs/healthsafetyguide/F1.htm. last modified 1/11/07. Accessed September 12, 2009.
6. Bloodborne pathogens and needlestick prevention. United States Department of Labor web site. Available at: http://www.osha.gov/SLTC/bloodbornepathogens/. last updated 1/22/09. Accessed September 10, 2009.
7. Ethylene oxide. OSHA Safety web site Available at: http://www.osha-safety.org/osha_ethylene_oxide.asp. 2003. Accessed August 25, 2009.
8. Hhs. What we do. U.S. Department of Health and Human Services web site Available at: http://www.hhs.gov/about/whatwedo.html. Accessed August 30, 2009.
9. About EPA. EPA: United States Environmental Protection Agency web site Available at: http://www.epa.gov/epahome/aboutepa.htm. Accessed August 25, 2009.
10. Klenzyme [package insert]. Steris Corporation, St. Louis (MO), February 2008. Available at: http://www.steris.com/produts/view.cfm?id=125. Accessed September 12, 2009.
11. Overview: FDA regulation of medical devices. Available at: http://www.qrasupport.com/FDA_MED_DEVICE.html. updated May 6, 2003 Accessed August 1, 2009.
12. Feigal D. Letter to hospitals re: changes in enforcement of FDA'S requirements on reprocessing of single-use devices. Available at: http://www.fda.gov/MedicalDevices/DeviceRegulationandGuidance/Reprocessing. September 25, 2001. Accessed August 25, 2009.
13. Ahca. Plans and construction. Available at: http://www.fdhc.state.fl.us/MCHQ/Plans/. Accessed September 13, 2009.
14. O'Keefe E. Federal eye report: VA facilities improperly sterilized colonoscopy equipment. Available at: http://www.voices.washingtonpost.com/federal-eye/2009/06an_internal_released_today_fin.html. Accessed August 27, 2009.
15. Bynum R. Army Times: VA hospital says sterilization issues fixed. Posted Wednesday August 26, 2009. Available at: http://www.armytimes.com/news/2009/08/ap_ga_va_hospital_082609/. Accessed August 27, 2009.

16. Department of Veterans Affairs Office of Inspector General. Healthcare inspection: use and reprocessing of flexible fiberoptic endoscopes at VA medical facilities. Report number 09-01784-146. June 16, 2009. Available at: http://www4.va.gov/oig/54/reports/VAOIG-09-01784-146.pdf. Accessed August 10, 2009.
17. The Joint Commission. Understand the quality of care measures. Available at: http://www.jointcommissionreport.org/background/qualityofcaremeasures.aspx. Accessed September 12, 2009.
18. American Professional Safety Trainers Alliance. Federal, state, and OSHA regulations, statutes, fines and penalties. Available at: http://www.apsta.org/laws-fines.html. Accessed August 11, 2009.
19. Centers for Medicare and Medicaid Services. Roadmap for implementing value driven healthcare in the traditional Medicare fee-for-service program. Available at: http://www.cms.hhs.gov/center/quality.asp. Accessed September 12, 2009.
20. Utah Administrative Code: rule R432-3. General Healthcare Facility Rules Inspection and Enforcement. Available at: http://www.rules.utah.gov/publicat/code/r432/r432-003.htm. Effective May 1, 2009. Accessed September 12, 2009.
21. Association of Perioperative Registered Nurses. Mission statement. In: Conner R, Blanchard J, Burlingame B, et al, editors. Perioperative standards and recommended practices. Denver (CO): Association of Perioperative Registered Nurses, Inc; 2009. p. 8.
22. The Association for the Advancement of Medical Instrumentation. Comprehensive guide to steam sterilization and sterility assurance in healthcare facilities. Arlington (VA): ANSI/AAMI ST79; 2006.
23. International Association of Healthcare Central Service Materiel Management. About us. Available at: http://www.iahcsmm.org/MemberServices/aboutUs.html. Accessed September 11, 2009.
24. Association for Professions in Infection Control and Epidemiology, Inc. Vision 2012: creating a preferred future. Available at: http://www.apic.org/AM/PrinterTemplate.cfm?Section=Member_Services. Accessed September 1, 2009.

Perioperative Sterilization and Disinfection: An Infection Prevention Perspective

Lynda D. Doell, MSN, RN

KEYWORDS

• Disinfection • Sterilization • Surgical site infections
• Contamination

Infection prevention in the perioperative arena requires collaboration between the perioperative nurse and the infection preventionist to "prevent surgical site infections and provide a safe environment for our patients and staff."[1] This article presents key concepts, processes, expected outcomes, possible barriers, and strategies to prevent surgical site infections (SSIs) and staff exposures in the perioperative health care setting from an infection prevention perspective.

Sterilization and disinfection are critical processes that are integral to patient and employee safety. Mastery of the principles of sterilization and disinfection and adherence to evidence-based best practice are core skills in perioperative nursing. Properly implemented, these processes can reduce the incidence of SSIs in patients and staff exposures to blood-borne pathogens.

SSIs impact patient safety and the quality and cost of care. According to the Society for Healthcare Epidemiology of America (SHEA), approximately 500,000 SSIs occur every year in the United States at a cost of $10 billion annually. Each patient with an SSI remains in the hospital an additional 7 to 10 days. In addition to pain and suffering, patients with SSIs may face additional surgery such as incision and drainage, removal of implants, percutaneous placement of drains, or insertion of antibiotic beads into the infected site. Seventy-seven percent of deaths among patients with SSIs are directly related to the infection.[2] The perioperative nurse is responsible for minimizing the risk for SSIs, because "the creation and maintenance of an aseptic environment have a direct influence on patient outcomes."[3]

Infection Prevention, Texas Health Presbyterian Hospital of Plano, 6200 West Parker Road, Plano, TX 75093-7914, USA
E-mail address: lyndadoell@texashealth.org

Perioperative Nursing Clinics 5 (2010) 355–371
doi:10.1016/j.cpen.2010.04.006
1556-7931/10/$ – see front matter © 2010 Published by Elsevier Inc.

Today, third-party payers may not reimburse facilities for avoidable adverse events such as SSIs. In 2008, the Centers for Medicare and Medicaid (CMS) implemented their pay-for-performance (P4P) program and no longer reimburse for SSIs such as mediastinitis after cardiac surgery, some orthopedic joint infections, and bariatric gastric procedure infections.[4,5]

KEY CONCEPTS AND PROCESSES
Culture of Safety

Patient safety, which relies heavily on infection prevention, is an expectation of consumers and organizations that protect consumers. Establishing a culture of safety is a multifaceted process that begins with senior management members, who must communicate organizational missions, visions, and values that support an environment where staff members feel safe in reporting near misses or errors that might harm, injure, or cause illness to patients, staff, or visitors. Organizational leaders, staff, subject matter experts, and frontline workers analyze errors and near misses to identify opportunities for improvement (OFIs), devise better practices, take appropriate action to correct or mitigate possible adverse events, and monitor the results.[6]

Accountability is a key concept in patient safety. Individuals working in the health care environment are held accountable for their actions and are responsible for implementing organizational policies and procedures, but at the same time, are not blamed for system failures.

"Workers' actions are held to the standard of a reasonable and careful person working under similar circumstances to avoid negligence, which is the failure to use such care."[6]

Healthcare executives, senior leaders, directors, and managers are responsible for ensuring that health care personnel are competent to perform their jobs.

Direct health care providers such as physicians, nurses, patient care technicians, and therapists and ancillary staff such as environmental services workers are responsible for using infection prevention practices. Facility leaders are responsible for holding staff members accountable for their actions regarding patient safety and infection prevention.[6] In a just culture, contributing factors are reviewed first, accountability determined, and then appropriate action is taken (Association of periOperative Registered Nurses [AORN] Position Statement on Creating A Patient Safety Culture). A just culture is not a blame-free environment, but one in which processes and individuals are evaluated, and there is an emphasis on creating an environment that minimizes the potential for human error.

The Nurse as Patient Advocate

AORN states that

"The safety of patients …is the primary responsibility of the perioperative registered nurse and…the patient–caregiver bond is founded on the patient's trust in the registered nurse and the surgical team."[7]

The Association for Professionals in Infection Control and Epidemiology (APIC) has a strong position statement on patient safety that states infection preventionists will emphasize prevention and promote zero tolerance for health care-associated infections and other adverse events.[8]

According to the 2008 Gallup Honesty and Ethics of Professionals Survey, nurses have the highest ranking for honesty and ethics for the seventh straight year, receiving a high or very high rating from 84% of the individuals who responded to the poll.[9] Infection preventionists working together with the perioperative team have opportunities to improve care and reduce adverse events for patients who have no family members or other personal advocates inside the closed environment of the surgical suite.

In the operating room, the staff members present are the patient's advocates. Nursing advocacy helps keep the patient safe when the patient is not able to speak for his or her own behalf. Nurses who follow policies and procedures, limit traffic in the operating room, participate in a time out, and put patients in the forefront of the perioperative environment act as patient advocates.[10] The American Nurses Association has an articulate description of ethical concerns and patient advocacy:

"By virtue of the nurse relationship and the altruistic nature of nursing, perioperative nurses have an inherent obligation to advocate for patients, themselves, and their colleagues (ie, the profession of nursing). This inherent obligation of advocacy is further articulated as the perioperative nurse's ethical obligation to provide, safe, professional, and ethical patient care. To be competent in providing ethical care, perioperative nurses must know how to make ethical decisions as a patient advocate while not compromising one's own moral conscience. Therefore, perioperative nurses must have a working knowledge of the Code of Ethics for Nurses and what is meant by ethical perioperative practice to not only strengthen the nurse's ethical and moral position in health care but also to ultimately better serve the interests of patients.[11]"

Infection preventionists join perioperative nurses in being champions for patient advocacy and being ethically obligated to support safe, professional, and ethical patient care.

Evidence-Based Practice

Evidence based practice (EBP) is "integrating individual clinical expertise with the best available external clinical evidence from systematic research."[12] Using EBP supports optimal patient care and should help clinicians align and integrate research, clinical guidelines, and outcomes assessments into their clinical practice.[13] The expected outcome is improved patient care that is quality-focused, safe, and cost-effective. Steps in identifying and using EBP include

- Forming a good clinical question
- Finding the evidence using effective search techniques
- Identifying resources for evidence-based practice including databases, E-journals, E-textbooks, and other Internet sites.[13]

Infection prevention and patient safety in the perioperative setting require a clean environment, trained staff, and surgical instruments that are "properly cared for, effectively reprocessed, and ready to use."[7] The perioperative nurse is responsible for implementing instrument processing recommendations and standards relevant to the operating room.[14] The infection preventionist collaborates with the perioperative staff to focus on prevention of adverse outcomes and SSIs and to investigate clusters or trends that may occur in either situation.

Communication

Communication is a critical skill for health care professionals and helps eliminate adverse and preventable patient outcomes.[15] Communication should be effective and clear. According to Gruber and Hartman

"Communication is indivisible from relationship building...and allows the nurse to effectively carry out his or her professional responsibilities."[15]

Registered nurses and other health care professionals rely on relationships for therapeutic and administrative effectiveness. Building professional relationships with patients and colleagues are the basis for performing professional responsibilities. In their study, listening, providing clear information, and effectively communicating decisions were the most important skills. Williams and Gosset identified four types of required nursing communication: communicating nursing assessments, encouraging clarification, encouraging questioning, and reassuring others.[16]

Policies and Procedures

Policies and procedures in the perioperative setting should minimally include

- Reducing modifiable patient risk factors
- Cleaning and disinfection of equipment and the environment
- Preparation and disinfection of the operative site and the hands of the surgical team
- Adherence to hand hygiene
- Traffic control in the operating room
- Adherence to standard principles of operating room asepsis
- Sterilizing equipment according to published guidelines and minimizing flash sterilization.[14]

Hand Hygiene

Hand hygiene is the single most important action individuals can take to prevent the spread of infection. In 1847, Dr Ignaz Semmelweis discovered that hand washing with a chlorinated-lime solution reduced the incidence deaths in women from childbed fever.[17] In the United States, rates of appropriate hand hygiene among trained health care workers are approximately 40%.[18] This low rate of compliance should not be acceptable to staff members working in health care.

Normal microbial flora on hands includes resident and transient bacteria. Resident flora are attached to deeper layers of the skin are more resistant to removal and less likely to be associated with infections. Transient bacteria that colonize the superficial layers of the skin are more likely to be removed by hand hygiene. Colonization is the presence of microorganisms in or on a host with growth and multiplication, but without tissue invasion or damage.[19] Health care workers acquire transient bacteria from direct contact with patients or direct contact with contaminated environmental surfaces. Their hands may be persistently colonized with bacteria flora from gram-negative and gram-positive bacteria or yeast. Transient flora are the bacteria most frequently associated with health care-associated infections. The use of appropriate hand hygiene reduces the number of transient bacteria on the hands. This process is important, because "improved hand hygiene practices have been associated with reduced health care-associated infection rates."[18]

In the perioperative environment, proper hand hygiene is critical to provide safe patient care and involves hand washing with soap and water, hand hygiene with alcohol hand rubs, and surgical hand antisepsis. Hand hygiene performed with soap and water or alcohol hand rub is designed to remove the transient bacteria from hands and reduce the resident bacteria. Surgical hand antisepsis is performed preoperatively and designed to eliminate transient bacteria and reduce resident bacteria before donning sterile gloves. The United States Food and Drug Administration (FDA) has regulatory oversight of hand antiseptic products. Surgical hand antisepsis in the operating room should "significantly reduce microorganisms on intact skin, contain a nonirritating, antimicrobial preparation, be broad-spectrum and fast-acting, and have a persistent effect."[20]

Contamination

Contamination is the presence of potentially infectious pathogenic microorganisms such as blood or other potentially infectious material (OPIM) on or in animate or inanimate objects.[21] In the perioperative setting, contamination may occur because of lack of appropriate hand hygiene or improper cleaning, disinfection, or sterilization of instruments or other equipment. Other sources of possible contamination include improper ventilation, insufficient disinfection or sterilization parameters, staff errors, and failure to follow existing policies and procedures.

Bioburden and Biofilm

Bioburden refers to degree of microbial load, which is the number of viable organisms contaminating an object. Blood, body fluids, and tissue are possible contaminants in the perioperative setting. Biofilm is a thin coating of biologically active organisms that have the ability to grow in water, water solutions, or in vivo and coat the surface of structures or objects. The organisms may be viable or nonviable, but the adherence to surfaces protects the organic matter and can prevent antimicrobial agents from reaching the cells. If cleaning is not done thoroughly, biofilm can remain in cracks or tape residue and contaminate equipment or surfaces.[22]

Cleanliness and Cleaning

Cleanliness is the absence of dust, soil, debris, bioburden, blood, or OPIM. The process of cleaning removes those substances from equipment, surfaces, and instruments in the perioperative environment using friction, detergent, and water to remove organic debris rather than kill microorganisms.[21] Cleaning must occur before disinfection and sterilization can be accomplished to reduce bioburden and remove foreign material that interferes with the sterilization process.[22]

The cleaning process for instruments used in surgery should be started in the operating room by wiping instruments with a damp cloth and rinsing or soaking instruments to prevent blood and tissue from drying on the instruments. After surgery, the instruments should be covered and taken to a dedicated decontamination area. Other products available to prevent debris from drying on instruments include foam, gels, and enzymatic sprays. The infection preventionist focuses on the appropriate cleaning, processing, inspection, and packaging of instruments before sterilization occurs to ensure quality and safe patient care.[14,23]

Disinfection

Before disinfection can be achieved, cleaning must be performed using water with detergents or enzymatic cleaners. Disinfectants are used only on inanimate objects.[14] Disinfection in the perioperative setting is based on the Spalding classifications of medical devices. Spalding classified devices into three categories: critical, semicritical, and noncritical. Critical items such as surgical instruments enter sterile body sites and require sterilization. Semicritical items such as laryngoscopes, respiratory therapy, and anesthesia equipment contact mucous membranes or nonintact skin and require high-level disinfection. High-level disinfection kills vegetative bacteria, tubercle bacteria, some spores, fungi, and lipid and nonlipid viruses. Noncritical items such as blood pressure cuffs, linens, and patient furniture contact intact skin and require low-level disinfection. Low-level disinfection kills most bacteria, some viruses, and some fungi.[22] The Environmental Protection Agency is responsible for regulating and registering chemical germicides used as sterilizers and disinfectants and works together with the FDA.[20]

Sterilization

Sterilization is a process that provides the highest level of assurance that surgical items are free of viable microbes. Sterilization is one of the most critical processes to prevent surgical site infections. Effective sterilization requires appropriate instrument cleaning and decontamination before sterilization occurs. Important steps in the sterilization process include instrument preparation, inspection, opening, unlocking, or disassembling, wrapping, or preparing containers, and paper or plastic pouches before sterilization. Health care staff should follow the manufacturer's guidelines for total container use and drying information.[24]

Flash Sterilization

Flash sterilization is "the process designated for the steam sterilization of patient care items for immediate use" and should not be considered as a routine method or used for the sterilization of implantable devices.[25] The Association of the Advancement of Medical Instrumentation (AAMI) provides criteria for flash sterilization that should be meticulously followed, documented, and monitored as a standard practice. Important steps in the flash sterilization process are cleaning, decontaminating, inspecting, correctly arranging instruments in the appropriate container, and placing instruments close to the point of use.[26] The Joint Commission has a focus on flash sterilization that traces the instruments from the time they leave one operating room to the time they return to another and verifies that staff members are using the appropriate personal protective equipment (PPE) and are able to articulate and follow the manufacturer's instructions for sterilization.[25] AORN recommends that flashed items be recorded and traceable back to a patient in the event of a biologic test failure. The flash sterilization process includes:

1. Cleaning
2. Decontamination
3. Inspecting
4. Correctly arranging instruments in the container or tray
5. Placing instruments close to where they will be used.[26]

Aseptic Technique

Aseptic or sterile technique is the purposeful prevention of transfer of organisms from one person to another by keeping the microbe count to the irreducible minimum.

Health care workers must meticulously adhere to aseptic technique in the perioperative environment to protect patients and staff and avoid transmitting microorganisms that can cause infections by direct or indirect contact. Examples of processes used to facilitate sterile technique are surgical hand antisepsis; donning of appropriate surgical attire such as sterile gowns and gloves, caps, masks, and eye protection; use of sterile drapes; and maintenance of a sterile field. Breaches or breaks in these processes increase the possibility of an adverse event for the patient such as SSIs and staff exposures to blood and body fluids.[27] The infection preventionist works closely with the perioperative staff to ensure that aseptic technique is not compromised to reduce the possibility of SSIs from biofilm, bioburden, contamination, or supplies that are expired or stored improperly.

Sterile Field

AORN defines the sterile field as the area around the site of the incision into tissue or the site of introduction of an instrument into the body orifice that has been prepared for the use of sterile supplies and equipment. The sterile field is maintained by rigorous adherence to aseptic practices by all individuals involved in surgical interventions.[28] Sterile supplies should be opened as close to the time of use as possible and used for one patient. Nonsterile equipment should be covered with sterile barrier materials before being introduced into the sterile field. The sterile field should be maintained and monitored continuously. Personnel in the operating room should move within and around the sterile field in a manner that maintains the sterile field. Staff members in the perioperative setting should wear appropriate scrubs, cover hair completely, avoid fleece material that may shed lint, and not leave the operating suite wearing dangling masks, shoe covers, or cover gowns.[29]

SSIs

Surgical procedures have varying risks depending on four clinical variables: the number of microorganisms contaminating the wound; the virulence of the microorganisms; the microenvironment of the wound including hematoma formation, necrosis, or presence of foreign material; and the integrity of the host defenses.[30] Wound classifications are: class 1 clean, class 2 clean-contaminated, class 3 contaminated, or class 4 dirty and infected.[31]

SSIs are classified as superficial incisional SSIs involving the skin and subcutaneous tissue, deep incisional SSIs involving the fascia and muscle, or organ space SSIs.[30] **Fig. 1** depicts a cross section of the abdominal wall using the Centers for Disease Control and Prevention's (CDC) classification for SSIs. Superficial infections must occur within 30 days after the operative procedure. Deep incisional or organ space SSIs must occur within 30 days after the operative procedure if no implant is left in place or 365 days after the operative procedure if an implant is used and the infection appears to be related to the operative procedure.[31] An example of a worksheet used for SSI data collection is seen in **Fig. 2**.

Surveillance

"Surveillance is a systematic method of collecting, consolidating, and analyzing data concerning the distribution and determinants of a given disease or event and then disseminating that information to those who can improve the outcomes."[32]

Surveillance should be based on sound epidemiologic and statistical principles, and it is essential for effective infection prevention. Surveillance supports the identification of risk factors for infection, implementation of risk reduction measures, and monitoring of the effectiveness of interventions.[31] "Surveillance is essential to identifying clusters, outbreaks, emerging infectious diseases and antibiotic-resistant organisms."[32] Surveillance programs should be aligned with quality improvement, patient safety, and cost effectiveness. Surveillance results should be reported to stakeholders using comparable data from similar organizations.

Infection preventionists perform surveillance on surgical patients for high-volume procedures, problem prone procedures, identified trends, or new procedures based on a risk assessment of the patient population. Readmitted patients' medical records also are reviewed. The data obtained are analyzed and compared with the National Healthcare Safety Network (NHSN) database for comparison.[33] Feedback is provided to key stakeholders.

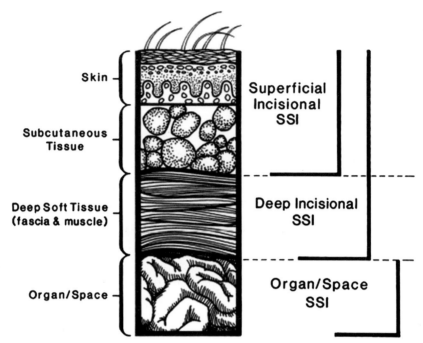

Skin

Subcutaneous
Tissue

Deep Soft Tissue
(fascia & muscle)

Organ/Space

Superficial
Incisional
SSI

Deep Incisional
SSI

Organ/Space
SSI

Fig. 1. Cross section of abdominal wall depicting surgical site infection classification. (*From* Horan TC, Gaynes RP, Martone WJ, et al. CDC definitions of nosocomial surgical site infections, 1992: a modification of CDC definitions of surgical wound infections. Infect Control Hosp Epidemiol 1992;13:606–8; with permission.)

In one study, laryngoscope handles were cultured using a polymerase chain reaction assay (PCR) after being cleaned and disinfected. The handles were cultured between cases when the room had been cleaned and the next case was ready to begin. Seventy five percent of the 40 handles cultured were positive for bacteria including *Staphylococcus*, *Bacillus*, *Streptococcus*, and *Enterococcus*.[34] Kable and Gibberd conducted a retrospective study on adverse events in five surgical procedures: cholecystectomy, transurethral resection of the prostate, hysterectomy, joint arthroplasty, and herniorrhaphy. They found an adverse event rate for postoperative infections of 41% (84 of 272 patients).[35] Tait and Tuttle conducted a random sample questionnaire for practicing anesthesiologists who were members of the American Society of Anesthesiologists (ASA). Forty percent of the respondents' rarely disinfected anesthesia working surfaces, and 19% reused syringes on more than one patient.[36] The contamination of anesthesia equipment can transmit bacterial or fungal infections from one patient to another. The infection preventionist investigates clusters or outbreak infections to identity possible breaks in techniques, process errors, or product contamination.

Product Selection

Product selection and availability are patient and staff safety concerns in the perioperative setting. Product selection should focus on functionality, safety, reliability, quality, and cost effectiveness.[37] Products selected should be used according to the

SSI Data Collection Form

NAME:	MR#	AGE:		ADM:		
		M F		DC:	READMIT DATE:	
PROCEDURE	DATE:	WND CLASS: CLEAN (I) CLEAN CONTAM (II) CONTAM (III) DIRTY (IV)				
	RM#:	ASA: 1 2 3 4 5	RISK:			
SURGERY TIME						
START	STOP	TIME	DURATION CUT POINT			
PROPHYLAXIS						
PRE	INTRA		IRRIGATION		POST	
TIME	TIME		TIME		TIME	
PERSONNEL						
SURGEON	ASSISTANTS		CIRCULATING		SCRUB	
ANESTHESIOLOGIST	ANESTHETIST		PERFUSION	HAIR REMOVAL		PREP
CULTURE	#1		#2		#3	
DATE:						
SITE						
ORGANISM(S)						
INFECTION TYPE Superficial Deep Organ space	HOSPITAL TREATMENT		HOME TREATMENT		COMMENTS	

Fig. 2. Surgical site infection worksheet.

manufacturer's recommendations, guidelines, and instructions. Staff members should be educated about new products before use. Monitoring and evaluation of the effectiveness of the product should be conducted. The infection preventionist scrutinizes product selection, availability, and use.

ISSUES IN PREVENTING INFECTION
Cleaning/Soaking

The infection preventionist monitors and reviews processes for soaking and cleaning of used instruments in the perioperative environment. Biofilm or bioburden that remains on instruments until after sterilization is a process error. Instruments with lumens or ports should be flushed to remove debris. Instruments should be taken

SIGNS/SYMPTOMS					
SUPERFICIAL INCISIONAL: Infection occurs 30 days after the operative procedure and involves only skin or subcutaneous tissue of the incision and at least one of the following:		**DEEP INCISIONAL SSI:** Infection occurs within 30 days after the operative procedure and no implants are left in place or within 1 year if implants are in place and the infection appears to be related to the operative procedure and infection involves deep soft tissues (e.g. facial and muscle layer) of the incision and at least one of the following is present:		**ORGAN/SPACE SSI:** Infection occurs within 30 days after the operative procedure and no implant is left in place or within 1 year if implant is in place and the infection appears to be related to the operative procedure and involves any part of the anatomy other than the incision opened or manipulated during the operative procedure, and at least one of the following is present:	
DATE		DATE		DATE	
	Purulent drainage from the superficial incision		Purulent drainage from the deep incision but not from the organ/space component of the surgical site		Purulent drainage from a drain that is placed through a stab wound in to the organ/space.
	Organisms isolated from an aseptically obtained culture of fluid or tissue from the superficial incision.		A deep incision spontaneously dehisces or is deliberately opened by a surgeon when the patient has a least one of the following signs or symptoms: fever (>38° c) localized pain or tenderness unless culture of the incision is negative.		Organism isolated from an especially obtained culture or fluid or tissue in the organ space
	At least one of the following signs or symptoms of infection, pain or tenderness, localized swelling, redness or heat *and* superficial incision is deliberately opened by surgeon and culture is negative		An abscess or other evidence of infection involving the deep incision is found on direct examination during operation or by histopathology or radiologic examination.		An abscess or other evidence of infection involving the organ space on direct examination during reoperation or by histopathology or radiologic examination.
	Diagnosis of superficial incision SSI by the surgeon or attending physician.		Diagnosis of deep incision SSI by surgeon or attending		Diagnosis of organ/space SSI by a surgeon or attending physician.

NOTE : Infection that involves both superficial and deep incision sites is classified as deep incisional SSI.

Occasionally an organ/space infection drains through the incision. Such infection generally does not involve reoperation and is considered a complication of the incision. It is therefore classified as a deep incisional SSI.

Fig. 2. (*continued*)

apart if applicable and stacked following manufacturer's recommendations. The perioperative staff acting as the patient advocate should ensure that instruments are cleaned, decontaminated, disinfected, and sterilized as appropriate before use following current standards, guidelines, policies, and procedures.[21]

Cleaning Supplies/Tools

Perioperative staff should use the appropriate supplies and tools to clean and decontaminate instruments and equipment. Cleaning, disinfection, and sterilizations should follow the manufacturer's guidelines. Manuals and instructions should be up-to-date and be specific to the instrument or equipment being used. When equipment is changed, replaced, or updated, using instructions from previous models or from prior manuals can cause errors that impact the cleanliness and lead to SSIs. For example, endoscopy equipment has ports and lumens that have special brushes and flushing devices per the manufacturer.[38] Using a cystoscopy brush on an endoscope may cause perforation or other damage, because the brush can have the wrong bristle strength, length, or configuration.

Drying

Instruments should be thoroughly dried. Moisture left on instruments promotes rust formation, can negatively impact the sterilization process, alters the moisture content of steam, and interferes with effective heating of instruments.[39] Wet packs allow microorganisms to enter the pack and contaminate sterilized items. Wet packs should be investigated and resolved to avoid adverse outcomes. The infection preventionist works in collaboration with the perioperative staff to investigate process concerns to avoid adverse events.

Multiple Drug Resistant Organisms

Contact isolation precautions are required for patients who are colonized or infected with multiple drug resistant organisms (MDROs) such as methicillin-resistant *Staphylococcus aureus* (MRSA), vancomycin-resistant *Enterococcus* (VRE), *Pseudomonas,* and *Acinetobacter*.[40] The route of transmission is from touching a contaminated person or object in the environment.[41] Nurses should communicate requirements for contact isolation precautions using the professional exchange report in electronic health record, by verbal communication, or using an established checklist of important patient information to communicate to other health care providers. Failure to communicate this information places the patients and health care workers at risk.

Ventilation

Operating rooms should be maintained at a positive pressure to adjacent areas with a minimum of 15 air exchanges per hour and a recommended rate of 20 to 25 air exchanges from the ceiling down to the floor. Doors to the operating room should remain closed. A properly functioning heating, ventilation, and air conditioning (HVAC) system reduces the risk of contamination to the sterile field and is essential to avoid infections.[42]

Environmental Cleaning

Accumulation of dust, debris, blood, body fluids, and other contaminants on environmental surfaces may be a source of contamination that can be transmitted on the hands of health care workers.[43] Dust has been found to contain human skin and hair, gram-negative bacteria such as *Staphylococcus,* fabric fibers, mold, fungi, insect parts, glove powder, and paper fibers. Perioperative nurses should assess cleanliness in the operating room and are responsible for verification that the surgical environment is clean working with the environmental services staff.[21] The infection preventionist also monitors cleanliness in the perioperative environment to reduce the possibility of SSIs.

Implants

The operating room environment is critical to minimize intraoperative contamination that can lead to infections in implanted devices.[44] Strategies to prevent intraoperative infections in patients with implants include traffic control in the operating room, minimizing microbial levels, maintaining positive air pressure, and ensuring compliance with air exchanges. Implant infections that occur within 365 days of the surgical procedure count as SSIs. A study done by physicians from the Mayo Clinic found that the pathogenesis of infections in prosthetic joint patients related to the presence of microorganisms in biofilm.[45] In a prospective cohort study done at a university medical center, researchers found an association (p = .008) between intraoperative wound contamination and the occurrence of a periprosthetic infection related to bacteria in the air in the operating room and the hands of surgical personnel or instruments.[46]

Flashing Instruments

No routine flashing should be used. Staff should ensure that flashed parameters meet requirements and that those requirements are documented. If one person starts the flash process, and another person removes the instruments, errors may occur. Staff should maintain logs for instruments that are flashed and monitor the reasons for flashing. Flashing should not be done for convenience, used to replace ordering sufficient instruments, or be used routinely for implants.[27]

Expired Supplies

Using out-of-date supplies can lead to adverse outcomes or infections. Package integrity must be maintained; supplies must be rotated to ensure using the oldest supplies first. Supply dates must be checked before use to identify outdated supplies, and packages and packs must be inspected for holes and tears before use to avoid using contaminated items. Staff should be vigilant and not assume supplies are useable without validating the date and package integrity. Any package or supply that is dropped on the floor is considered contaminated and should not be used for patient care unless the supply can be appropriately recleaned, disinfected, and sterilized according to the manufacturer's instructions for use.

Storage of Supplies

Sterile supplies should be stored properly to maintain sterility until the product is used. Sterile supplies should be appropriately packaged and labeled and include the date of sterilization. Outside shipping containers should not be allowed in the storage area. Stored items should be rotated so that the oldest supplies are used first. The shelf life of sterile supplies is event-related. The sterile supply may be used as long as the sterility has not been compromised by moisture, holes in the packaging, excessive humidity, dust, or other potential contamination.[46] Linen should be stored in covered carts to avoid contamination. Supplies should not be stored closer than 18 in from the ceiling or on carts or racks without solid bottom shelves to avoid contamination from splashes while mopping the floor.

Reprocessing Bronchoscopes and Endoscopes

Reprocessing of scopes is critical to infection prevention. Reprocessing should follow the manufacturer's recommendations and include appropriate cleaning, leak testing, flushing, disinfection, drying, and storage for that make and model of the instrument. Foam cases should not be used for storage or transport of scopes inside a facility, because foam cannot be cleaned. Foam cases may be used to transport scopes outside facilities for repairs. When the scope returns from repair, the instrument should be reprocessed before use. The American Society for Gastrointestinal Endoscopy (ASGE) identified stringent reprocessing of endoscopes after use as the single best protection against patient-to-patient transmission of pathogenic microorganisms. The inherent complexity of the instruments with their long narrow lumens, flexible joints, multiple channels, openings, and values pose significant reprocessing challenges.

Reprocessing requires meticulous cleaning and high-level disinfection or sterilization of internal channels, external surfaces, openings (ports), valves, and caps. Accessory equipment used to biopsy, brush, or cut tissue must be cleaned and sterilized or discarded if disposable.[47]

Documentation

The AORN Perioperative Standards and Recommended Practices have a list of 24 requirements for perioperative documentation in the patient's medical record.[48] The infection preventionist uses this critical documentation during an epidemiologic investigation and case review for a possible SSI. Infection preventionists investigate SSIs by reviewing the patient's medical record for important documentation that verifies and validates the care that was provided. Perioperative staff should document lines, drains, catheters, sutures, dressings, equipment used, skin preparations, the method of hair removal, antibiotic timing, and other details in the patient's medical record. The intraoperative nurse's notes are helpful to the infection preventionist during surveillance for SSIs.

Loaner Instruments

Instruments brought into operating room from outside the facility should be examined, cleaned, decontaminated, and reprocessed before use following the written instructions of the manufacturer. Perioperative staff should treat loaner instruments as nonsterile, because possible variations in the cleaning, decontamination, disinfection, sterilization, and proper storage of the instruments are unknown and could have occurred. Patients are not safe if the surgical instruments used on them during their surgical procedures are assumed to be sterile without verification.

PREVENTION STRATEGIES
Infection Prevention Round

Infection prevention rounds in the perioperative setting are important for monitoring and reviewing patient safety, quality, and data collection. The infection preventionist collects data, previews outcome measures, and provides feedback to key stakeholders. Rounding should include observations of health care staff for compliance with hand hygiene, maintenance of the sterile field, cleanliness in the perioperative environment, review of supplies and storage areas, and discussion with staff to identify areas of concern. Rounding results should be shared with the staff and reported to oversight committees and senior leaders. Results that require correction or improvement should be aligned with action plans that have a definite time frame for correction. Best practices and successes also should be shared. Because the infection preventionist works outside the perioperative environment rounding provides critical information to support patient safety, reduction of SSIs, and quality care. The infection preventionist's role is to assist and support the perioperative staff to provide quality and safe patient care and to promote staff safety.

Monitoring

Infection preventionists should review and monitor policies and procedures in the perioperative setting for accuracy and compliance. Polices should be evidence-based, reflect appropriate current recommendations and requirements, and be followed by the staff. Tools are available to help participants analyze the data collected. Failure mode and effects analysis (FMEA), root cause analysis (RCA), force field analysis, and the VALUE model (validate, analyze, list improvements, use improvements, and evaluate actions) are helpful to identify OFIs. Another tool is a safe choices algorithm that leaders may use to coach and mentor staff.[8] Successful solutions and lessons learned are shared with other departments and across hospitals in a system to drive improved outcomes of care. An example of a force field analysis is seen in **Fig. 3**.

MindTools

Essential skills for an excellent career

The Internet's Most
Visited Career Skills Resource

Force Field Analysis Worksheet

- For instructions on Force Field Analysis, visit www.mindtools.com/rs/ForceField.
- For more business leadership skills visit www.mindtools.com/rpages/HowtoLead.htm.

Forces FOR change	Score		Change proposal		Forces AGAINST change	Score
>SSIs with MRSA	5				Staff knowledge deficit	4
6 are joint implants	5				Resistance to change	5
Patient dissatisfaction	4		Compare rates with NHSN		Use of contact isolation	4
Loss of revenue	3		Do individual case review		No prior MRSA screen	5
Increased length of stay	3		Consider patient decolonization		2 day lab result time	3
Possible transmission	4		Find physician champion		Unaware of cost issues	3
			Report data and summary to key stakeholders			
			Use rapid PCR for MRSA with 2 hour turnaround time			
TOTAL	24				TOTAL	24

For new tools like this every two weeks, subscribe to the free Mind Tools newsletter:
http://www.mindtools.com/subscribe.htm.

Fig. 3. Force field analysis (*Courtesy of* MindTools. Copyright © MindTools Ltd., 2006–2009.).

The National Healthcare Safety Network (NHSN), established in 2005, is a voluntary Internet-based surveillance system managed by the Division of Healthcare Quality Promotion at the CDC. Enrollment in NHSN is available to health care facilities in the United States. The NHSN provides criteria for surveillance of health care-associated infections

"resulting from an adverse reaction to the presence of an infectious agent or toxin. The infection cannot be present or incubating at the time of admission to the acute care setting."[33]

Once an infection is identified by the infection preventionist, the specific type of infection is determined by using the NHSN criteria that allows for comparing rates with other acute care facilities, because NHSN aggregates surveillance data into a single national database. Colonization and inflammation that result from tissue response to injury or stimulation by noninfectious agents are not considered infections. SSIs are defined as infections occurring up to 30 days after surgery or up to 365 days after surgery if the patient receives an implant during surgery.[33]

Surgical Care Improvement Project

The Surgical Care Improvement Project (SCIP), which began in 2003, is an extension of the Surgical Infection Prevention Collaborative (SIP) started by the CMS in 2002. SIP focused on appropriate antibiotic timing, administration, and discontinuation for seven specific procedures: abdominal and vaginal hysterectomies, hip and knee arthroplasties, cardiac surgery, vascular surgery, and colorectal surgery. Three additional evidence-based measures have been added. Hair should not be removed from the operative site unless the hair interferes with the operative procedure. If hair removal is required, a hair clipper or depilatory should be used. Razors should not be used to shave hair at the operative site. Patients undergoing cardiac surgery should have blood glucose levels controlled during the immediate postoperative period. Patients undergoing colorectal surgery should have normothermia maintained during the perioperative period.[2]

SUMMARY

The infection prevention perspective places the safety and well-being of the patient and the staff as the central focus of each action taken. Strong collaboration efforts between the professional staff in the perioperative environment and the infection preventionist should be directed to "prevent surgical site infections and provide a safe environment for our patients and staff."[1] This article presented key concepts, processes, expected outcomes, possible barriers, and strategies to prevent staff exposures and SSIs in the perioperative health care setting from an infection prevention perspective. Important lessons learned are to never assume processes are always done correctly. The patient's life depends on verification of processes and not on assumptions. The perioperative and infection prevention staff should adopt a zero tolerance for SSIs and continue to be strong patient advocates.

REFERENCES

1. AORN. AORN guidelines and guideline statements. Patient safety culture. Denver (CO): AORN, Incorporated; 2009. p. 237–41.
2. Anderson DJ, Kaye KS, Classen D, et al. Strategies to prevent surgical site infections in acute care hospitals. Infect Control Hosp Epidemiol 2008;29(Suppl 1): S51.

3. Gunn M. AORN, APIC set tone of collaboration an international infection prevention week. Available at: http://www.aorn.org/news/managers/october2009issue/iipw/. Accessed October 15, 2009.

4. Pear SM, Williamson TH. The RN first assistant: an expert resource for surgical site infection prevention. AORN J 2009;89(6):1093.

5. Association of periOperative Registered Nurses (AORN). Recommended practices for perioperative nursing. Recommended practices for sterilization in the perioperative practice setting. Denver (CO): AORN, Incorporated; 2009. p. 647.

6. Seavey R. The need for educated staff in sterile processing: patient safety depends on it. Perioperative Nursing Clinics 2009;4:181.

7. Association of periOperative Registered Nurses. Standards, recommended practices and guidelines. Position statement on patient safety. Denver (CO): Association of Perioperative Registered Nurses, Incorporated; 2007. p. 398–400.

8. Murphy DM. Patient safety. Association for Professionals in Infection Control and Epidemiology (APIC). Washington, DC: APIC, Incorporated; 2005. p. 12-1–12-5.

9. Sand L. Nurses shine, bankers slump in ethics ratings. Available at: http://www.gallup.com/poll/112264/nurses-shine-while-bankers-slump-ethics-ratings.aspx. Accessed October 15, 2009.

10. Beyea SC. Patient advocacy nurses keeping patients safe. Available at: http://findarticles.com/p/articles/mi_m0FSL/is_5_81/ai_n13793213/. Accessed September 12, 2009.

11. The ANA code of ethics and AORN's interpretive statements. Available at: http://periopnursing.theclinics.com/article/S1556-7931(08)00041-7/fulltest?Submitt. Accessed September 14, 2009.

12. Sackett DL. Evidence-based practice. Available at: http://www.med.yale.edu/library/nursing/education/ebhc.html. Accessed September 12, 2009.

13. DeBourgh GA. Evidence-based practice. Available at: http://www.med.yale.edu/library/nursing/education/ebhc.html. Accessed September 14, 2009.

14. Mullaney K. Sterilization and disinfection in the operating room. Perioperative Nursing Clinics 2008;3:127–34.

15. Grubee M, Hartman R. Don't overlook communication competence. Nurs Manag 2007;38(3):12–4.

16. Williams CA, Gosset MT. Nursing communication: advocacy for the patient or physician? Clin Nurs Res 2001;10(3):332–40.

17. Centers for Disease Control and Prevention. Wash your hands. Available at: http://www.cdc.gov/Features/Handwashing/. Accessed September 15, 2009.

18. Underwood MA. Hand hygiene. Washington, DC: APIC, Incorporated; 2005. p. 19-1–19-6.

19. CDC. Guideline for hand hygiene in health-care settings. MMWR Morb Mortal Wkly Rep 2002;51(RR 16):2.

20. AORN. AORN recommended practices for perioperative nursing. Recommended Practices for Surgical Hand Antisepsis/Hand Scrub. Denver (CO): AORN, Incorporated; 2009. p. 309.

21. AORN. AORN recommended practices for perioperative nursing. Environmental Cleaning. Denver (CO): AORN, Incorporated; 2009. p. 449–50.

22. AORN. AORN recommended practices for perioperative nursing. High Level Disinfection. Denver (CO): AORN, Incorporated; 2009. p. 579–90.

23. AORN. AORN recommended practices for perioperative nursing. Sterilization. Denver (CO): AORN, Incorporated; 2009. p. 647.

24. Clement L. An infection control practitioner's survival guide to understanding sterile processing. Mentor (OH): Steris Corporation; 2007.

25. The Joint Commission (TJC). Steam sterilization: update on THC's position. Available at: http://www.jointcommission.org/library/whatsnew/steam_sterilization.htm. 2009. Accessed October 20, 2009.
26. Mageri MA. Flash sterilization revisited. Perioperative Nursing Clinics 2008;3:1.
27. Decastro MG, Iwamoto P. Aseptic technique. Washington, DC: APIC, Incorporated; 2005. p. 20-1–20-3.
28. AORN. AORN recommended practices for perioperative nursing. Sterile field. Denver (CO): AORN, Incorporated; 2009. p. 323.
29. Xve Y. Surgical site infection: operating room environment controls. Available at: http://swtuopproxy.museglobal.com/MuseSessionID=6631a6d0afc7659aa9e03b3cbc7bd0c. Accessed September 12, 2009.
30. Janelle J, Howard RJ, Fry D. Surgical site infections. Washington, DC: APIC, Incorporated; 2005. p. 23-1–23-9.
31. Horan TC, Gaynes RP, Martone WJ, et al. CDC definitions of nosocomial surgical site infections, 1992: a modification of CDC definitions of surgical wound infections. Infect Control Hosp Epidemiol 1992;13:606–8.
32. Arias KM. Surveillance. Washington, DC: APIC, Incorporated; 2005. p. 3-1–3-7.
33. National Healthcare Safety Network. Report 2008. Available at: http://www.cdc.gov.nhsn/. Accessed September 14, 2008.
34. Call TR, Auerbach FJ, Riddell SW, et al. Nosocomial contamination of laryngoscope handles: challenging current guidelines. Anesthesia and Analgesia 2009;109(2):479–83. Available at: http://www.anesthanalg.org. Accessed October 18, 2009.
35. Kable A, Gibberd R. Adverse events in five surgical procedures. Clin Govern Int J 2009;14(2):145–55.
36. Tait AR, Tuttle DB. Preventing perioperative transmission of infection: a survey of anesthesia practice. Anesth Analg 1995;80:764–9.
37. AORN. AORN recommended practices for perioperative nursing. Product selection. Denver (CO): AORN, Incorporated; 2009. p. 387.
38. ASGE issues updated infection control guidelines for gastrointestinal endoscopy. Healthc Purch News 2008;32(7):32.
39. AORN. AORN recommended practices for perioperative nursing. Care of instruments. Denver (CO): AORN, Incorporated; 2009. p. 620.
40. Williams TN, Haas JP. Multidrug-resistant pathogen: implementing contact isolation in the operating room. Perioperative Nursing Clinics 2008;3:149–53.
41. Siegel JD, Rhinehart E, Jackson M, et al. Management of multidrug-resistant organisms in healthcare settings. The Healthcare Infection Control Practices Advisory Committee, 2006. Am J Infect Control 2007;35:S165–93.
42. AORN. AORN recommended practices for perioperative nursing. HVAC. Denver (CO): AORN, Incorporated; 2009. p. 421.
43. AORN. AORN recommended practices for perioperative nursing. Cleaning. Denver (CO): AORN, Incorporated; 2009. p. 439.
44. Montero JA. Implants. Washington, DC: APIC, Incorporated; 2005. p. 42.1–42.7.
45. Patel R, Asmon DR, Hanssen AD. The diagnosis of prosthetic joint infection. Clin Orthop Relat Res 2005;437:55–8.
46. Knobben BA, Engelsmo Y, Neut D, et al. Intraoperative contamination influences wound discharge and periprosthetic infection. Clin Orthop Relat Res 2006;452:236–41.
47. Stricof RL. Endoscopy: APIC Test of infection control and epidemiology. 2nd edition. Washington, DC: APIC Incorporated; 2005.
48. AORN. AORN recommended practices for perioperative nursing. Documentation. Denver (CO): AORN, Incorporated; 2009. p. 488.

Reprocessing and Remanufacturing: A Twenty-First Century Perspective

Liz Stoneman, RN, BSN

KEYWORDS

• Clinical sustainability • Reprocessing • Remanufacturing

The future of health care depends on clinical sustainability, which includes delivering best patient outcomes; being responsive to changes in the health care environment; and incorporating the latest techniques, advances, and equipment. The perioperative nurse professional is a key component in the facility's efforts to achieve clinical sustainability.

Clinicians and the nation are aware that health care is responsible for the inefficient consumption of massive amounts of resources, and there are frequently reminders of the detrimental impact of these inefficiencies on the quality of health, cost of health care, and the environment. Today, improving the health care system and exploring environmental initiatives are no longer abstract goals, but rather are vital and immediate necessities. Success is no longer dependent solely on patient outcomes, but also requires cost-effectiveness and efficiency in achieving those outcomes. Initiatives that promote clinical sustainability have emerged as the cornerstone of responsible hospital practice and leadership. This article provides a twenty-first century perspective on the responsible reprocessing of single-use devices (SUDs), which has emerged as a safe, regulated, and controlled option for cost-effective and efficient patient care.

Maintaining clinical sustainability requires frequent assessment of hospital resources and practices to ensure the best, the most efficient, and the most cost-effective outcomes for patients, the health care delivery system, and the environment. Perioperative nurses are a driving force in pursuit of practices that deliver responsible patient care and produce optimal patient outcomes. The best professionals consistently scan their environment for opportunities to improve practice and increase value.

Many hospitals are adapting to current demands for efficiency and effectiveness by partnering with industry in creative ways that drive sustainability. The remanufacturing and reprocessing of carefully selected SUDs is one such successful partnership.

Ascent Healthcare Solutions, 10232 South 51st Street, Phoenix, AZ 85044, USA
E-mail address: lstoneman@ascenths.com

Perioperative Nursing Clinics 5 (2010) 373–375
doi:10.1016/j.cpen.2010.05.003
1556-7931/10/$ – see front matter © 2010 Elsevier Inc. All rights reserved.

Appropriately reprocessed and remanufactured devices meet the key quality and sustainability imperatives of safety, efficiency, and cost-effectiveness.

The motivation for remanufacturing and reprocessing is simple: single-use medical devices are expensive assets, not trash. Although most SUDs cannot be used again and must be thrown away or recycled, some meet the stringent criteria for reprocessing. With discrimination and clinical and technical expertise some SUDs can be remanufactured to perform at their original level for one or more additional uses.

Safety is the primary concern when evaluating medical devices. Ensuring that the quality of remanufactured and reprocessed medical devices is equivalent to the quality of the originals is essential. Third-party remanufacturing and reprocessing has been around for a long time and has evolved into a strong component of clinical sustainability for health care facilities. The process has evolved under the close scrutiny of the Food and Drug Administration (FDA), as mandated by Congress and reviewed by the Government Accountability Office. Approved third-party remanufacturers and reprocessors deliver the highest quality and safety standards available today in the medical device industry.

Selecting SUDs appropriate for reprocessing and remanufacturing is integral to sustainability, and credible commercial reprocessors are very selective in the products they accept for remanufacturing. Only 2% to 5% of all SUDs are cleared by the FDA for limited and controlled reuse. Selection criteria include the complexity of the device and the risk associated with its use. Reprocessing requires complete disassembly and reassembly, so highly complex devices are usually not acceptable.

Risk is determined by the FDA classification of medical devices (Class I, Class II, and Class III), which is based on the potential for patient injury if the device fails or is misused. Class I devices (eg, blood pressure cuffs and thermometers) are often simple in design and present minimal potential for patient injury. Class II devices (eg, endoscopes, surgical drills, saws, and insufflators) include those whose misuse, failure, or absence with no replacement available would have a significant impact on patient care, but would not be likely to cause serious injury or death. Class III devices are considered "high risk" (eg, intracardiac pacemakers and implants) and would have potentially disastrous consequences as a result of misuse or failure. Any Class III device, because of the risk for patient harm, would be a poor choice for reprocessing. Currently, no Class III implantable devices are remanufactured or reprocessed.

The Association for the Advancement of Medical Instrumentation's Technical Information Report entitled "A compendium of processes, materials, test methods, and acceptance criteria for cleaning reusable medical devices," which was circulated to ballot committee and any public reviewers for final review before final submission, determines the methodology for performing cleaning validations. The report was compiled by representatives from the FDA, testing facilities, academia, hospitals, and representatives of the medical device industry. It identifies the indicators for cleanliness during cleaning validations.

In establishing a validation process, the company establishes "worst case" contamination to ensure that the reprocessing and remanufacturing process is effective for even the dirtiest devices. The company first analyzes a large number of "native" devices, devices that have been used clinically. By measuring the amounts of bioburden and organic soil residuals on these native devices, the company can establish the maximum amount of soil that can be expected on such a device on arrival. Next, the company challenges the devices with an artificial soil formulated to most closely mimic the tissue and debris the device may be exposed to during clinical use. For instance, phaco tips used in cataract surgery are soiled with artificial "eyeball" soil and electrophysiology catheters are soiled with artificial blood. The soil is contaminated with a minimum of 10^6 spores of *Geobacillus stearothermophilus*, an organism incredibly resistant to chemical sterilants and disinfectants. During this soiling process, devices are taken through a full range of motion numerous times to ensure that internal lumens or mated surfaces are exposed to contamination, then "powered up" (ie, subjected to conditions that are most difficult to clean, such as fixed, dried bioburden).

Reprocessing and remanufacturing is highly regulated and takes place in sophisticated manufacturing facilities. Reprocessing SUDs or "disposable" devices involves cleaning, disinfecting, sterilizing, and testing the function of each product according to FDA regulation, so that it can be safely used again. Remanufacturing of a "finished product" (used device) occurs after the product has been dismantled to its component parts and properly cleaned and disinfected. Each part is then inspected, repaired, refurbished, or replaced, and the device is reconstructed using only components that have passed all inspections. It is then tested and sterilized.

Substantial equivalence is established by ensuring that the intended use, design, energy used or delivered, materials, performance, safety, effectiveness, labeling, biocompatibility, standards, and other applicable characteristics of a remanufactured product are equivalent to a new one. The FDA "clears" a device for sale when it has established that the device is substantially equivalent through a comprehensive process of scientific review. There are no exceptions to the FDA's review process.

The reprocessing industry has evolved significantly since the reuse of SUD-labeled devices was first regulated in the early 1990s. The industry has changed how hospitals look at "single-use" devices. Practices have evolved to ensure that hospitals can safely participate in reuse while improving procurement practices and reducing environmental harm.

Reprocessing of Single-Use Devices: Do the Benefits Outweigh the Potential Dangers?

Michelle R. Tinkham, RN, BSN, PHN, MS, CNOR, CLNC, RNFA

KEYWORDS

- Single-use device • Patient safety
- Reprocessing • Perioperative nurse

Until 1948, when the first single-use device (SUD) was created, medical supplies were meant to be reused.[1] It was thought that reprocessing of these items was safe until patient injuries began to surface, many causing death. As a result, in the 1970s, original equipment manufacturers (OEMs) began labeling their devices, especially those containing plastics, as single use only.[1] As time went on and the costs associated with providing patient care increased, many health care facilities turned to reprocessing once again as a method of saving money; reprocessing often saved several hundreds of thousands of dollars a year.

There were again many reports of patient injury associated with these reprocessed devices due to improper cleaning or malfunctions, even though Food and Drug Administration (FDA) regulations to ensure patient safety were not in place until 2000.[2] A decade later, this debate is ongoing. The benefits of reprocessing SUDs are clear, but the potential for patient harm is hazy. There are substantial reasonable arguments that support both sides—the positive financial impact and the potential for patient injury—making the decision more difficult. OEMs state that the safety of reprocessed items cannot be guaranteed, especially because reprocessing companies do not have access to original product designs; the reprocessing companies state there is no evidence showing that appropriately reprocessed SUDs are less safe than their new counterparts. As a result, it is imperative for perioperative nurses to educate themselves regarding the FDA recommendations for reprocessing techniques and what should and should not be reprocessed.

7450 Northrop, Dr #38 Riverside, CA 92508, USA
E-mail address: Michelle.Tinkham@SBCglobal.net

Perioperative Nursing Clinics 5 (2010) 377–381
doi:10.1016/j.cpen.2010.04.007   **periopnursing.theclinics.com**
1556-7931/10/$ – see front matter © 2010 Elsevier Inc. All rights reserved.

WHAT CAN BE REPROCESSED?

According to the FDA, as of 2005, 229 items were approved for reprocessing; 78 were specifically for surgery and new items are added frequently (**Table 1**). The list of items is frequently updated and can be accessed at the FDA Web site (http://www.fda.gov/MedicalDevices/DeviceRegulationandGuidance/ReprocessingofSingle-UseDevices/default.htm). Just because the FDA has approved a device for reprocessing, however, does not mean that all third-party reprocessors reprocess that item. For instance, some companies do not reprocess class III medical devices due to the additional risks involved with these items.[3] Class I items, such as dressings, are considered lowest risk. Class II items are medium risk, and class III are the highest risk and include implantable devices, such as cardiac valves.[4] It is important for perioperative nurses to be aware of which items their facilities reprocess so these items may be collected or discarded appropriately.

In most cases, there are two collection types: opened and unused or expired items, and items that have been used but are appropriate for reprocessing. These two item types should not be mixed. Pharmaceutical items and items that break down after expiration, such as latex gloves, should not be reprocessed.[4] When in doubt about a specific item, contact the sterile processing department to determine if the item is resterilized in house, or contact the third-party reprocessing company if the item is reprocessed off site. All third-party reprocessors should have a list of the approved reprocessing services they offer for which they have received 510(k) clearance from the FDA. This list can often be accessed on a company's Web site.

Table 1	
Examples of approved reprocessed surgical items	
Device	**Class**
Endoscopic guide wire	II
Endoscopic trocars	II
Breast implant sizers	Unclassified
Implantable clip	II
Electrosurgical devices	II
Scalpel blades	I
Bits, burrs, and blades	I
Dermatome	I
Pneumatic tourniquet	I
Laser fibers	II
Percutanous biopsy forceps	III
Intraaortic balloon system	III
Angiography catheter	II
Electrophysiology catheters	II, III
Compression sleeves	II
Laproscopic instruments	II
Arthroscopic shavers, burrs	II

From FDA list of single-use devices known to be reprocessed or considered for reprocessing. Available at: http://www.fda.gov/medicaldevices/deviceregulationandguidance/reprocessingofSingle-UseDevices/ucm121218.htm. Accessed April 4, 2010. *Data from* Cohoon BD. Reprocessing single-use medical devices. AORN J 2002;75(3):557–67.

THE BENEFITS OF REPROCESSING

There are many benefits to reprocessing SUDs. In-house and off-site reprocessing by approved companies can mean substantial cost savings for health care facilities. Reprocessing also represents a form of recycling that not only helps facilities with the cost of waste disposal but also has community and environmental benefits. Reprocessing is especially beneficial considering the large number of appropriately salvageable items that otherwise would be wasted if not reprocessed. Third-party reprocessed items are often sold back to facilities at half the original cost; when reprocessing is done in facilities themselves, the savings can be as high as 90%.[5]

In August 2000, the FDA issued a guidance statement regarding reprocessing SUDs. Before this time, many hospitals and third-party companies did not meet these standards for reprocessing[4]; since August 2000, this is no longer the case. The FDA has spent years researching the reprocessing of SUDs and conducting compliance reviews. The FDA inspects third-party reprocessors approximately every 2 years and inspects OEMs every 4 years to be sure they are meeting the prescribed standards.[4]

In addition, the FDA investigates all reports of patient injury that involve a reprocessed SUD. Although there have been many reports over the years, research has found that most of the claims of patient injury were inconclusive. As a result, the FDA believes there is "reasonable assurance of safety and effectiveness of reprocessed SUDs for patients."[4] In 2006, the FDA made a public statement that it believes "that reprocessed SUDs that meet FDA's regulatory requirements are as safe and effective as a new device."[4] If these products are viewed by the FDA as safe and equivalent to a new item, it is not unreasonable for hospitals to agree. As a result, many facilities feel there is no need for additional informed consent before using reprocessed SUDs, because the consent is for a proposed procedure, not for what equipment is used.[5] Facilities also believe there is no need to charge patients a different price for reprocessed and new items because they are deemed equivalent.[5]

RISKS ASSOCIATED WITH REPROCESSING

Any item that is reprocessed must be manufactured in a way that allows the product to be completely disassembled and cleaned properly. There must be information available on proper cleaning and sterilization agents, instructions for assembly and disassembly, and proper water temperature exposure to ensure that all bioburden can be destroyed.[6] This information may be difficult to acquire because many OEM companies claim that reprocessors do not have access to their proprietary product specifications.[7] This lack of manufacturer instructions may also make it difficult to properly test items to ensure they are equivalent to the original products. Even when this information is available, there are many other potential risks associated with reuse. Alterations in equipment design integrity may adversely affect strength or performance, causing patient injury. Inadequate cleaning may lead to infections. Absorption of cleaning agents may have a toxic effect on patients.[6] Many OEMs have stated they have performed testing of reprocessed versions of their products and have found many issues. For example, Smith & Nephew stated it found contamination, compromised packaging, and product damage to its products after reprocessing.[8] Some manufacturers have published position statements regarding reprocessing of their devices.

OEMs are not the only ones who are hesitant regarding the reprocessing of SUDs. A study in 2002 found that 82% of nurses and 71% of physicians would not want reprocessed SUDs used during their own surgeries.[8] There are several states and patient advocacy groups that have proposed legislation that addresses liability, patient billing, and patient consent when reprocessed items are used.[8] As of 2006, third-party reprocessors were required to label their reprocessed items so they are easily distinguishable compared with the original. Due to poor tracking and reporting processes within facilities, however, some patient injuries may not be linked to a reprocessed item. As a result, many feel that the FDA has not done enough to ensure patient safety before approving these items. Few data have been published in the past 5 years regarding reprocessing of SUDs despite the continued controversy.

REGULATIONS AND STANDARDS

Ensuring that FDA criteria are met is one method of promoting patient safety in reprocessing. There are three essentials to consider before reprocessing, all of which are supported by the Association of Operating Room Nurses (AORN) guidance statement[9] for the reuse of SUDs:

1. If a device cannot be properly cleaned, it cannot be reprocessed.
2. If a reprocessed device cannot be proved functionally equal to its original counterpart, it cannot be reprocessed.
3. If a device cannot be resterilized properly, it cannot be reprocessed.

The FDA regulations attempt to ensure that hospitals and third-party reprocessors are reprocessing only those items that meet these criteria. The FDA requires reprocessors to register, list all items they are approved to reprocess, label items as reprocessed (**Figs. 1** and **2**), and track and report problems to MedWatch.[1]

After more than a decade of discussion, reprocessing of SUDs is still under public scrutiny and the controversy is often sensationalized by media reports with little supporting evidence. In today's environment of financial challenge, health care facilities need to be able to provide safe patient care as cost effectively as possible. The proper reprocessing of SUDs is one means of reducing the cost of patient care safely. If facilities are going to reprocess SUDs on site or through a third-party reprocessing company, the facilities must do everything possible to ensure that FDA requirements are met and that they are providing a safe and effective product to the patients who entrust their lives to those facilities. It is the facilities' responsibility to decide which

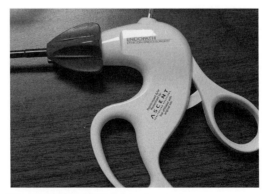

Fig. 1. Reprocessed item labeled with third-party name.

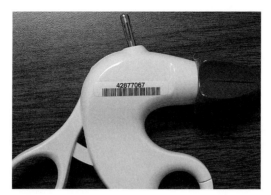

Fig. 2. Sample of tracking system used by third-party reprocessor.

items are reprocessed and it is perioperative nurses' responsibility to educate themselves about reprocessing and what can and what cannot be reprocessed according to facility policy, to understand the risks, and to follow protocol so that they may provide fiscally sound, environmentally friendly, and safe patient care.

REFERENCES

1. Cohoon BD. Reprocessing single-use medical devices. AORN J 2002;75(3): 557–67.
2. Schraag J. SUD reprocessing update. Retrieved January 12, 2010. From Infection Control Today: Available at: http://www.infectioncontroltoday.com/. Accessed January 12, 2010.
3. Ascent Healthcare Solutions. Reprocessing services list. Retrieved April 2, 2010. Available at: www.ascenths.com/docs/MARK-1237_Rev_BE_Reprocessing_ Services_List.pdf. Accessed April 2, 2010.
4. Schultz D. News & events: single-use devices (SUDs). Retrieved August 23, 2009. From FDA: Available at: http://www.fda.gov/NewsEvents/Testimony/ucm110940. htm. Accessed August 23, 2010.
5. Dunn D. Reprocessing single-use devices—the ethical dilemma. AORN J 2002; 75(5):989–99.
6. Dunn D. Reprocessing single-use devices—the equipment connection. AORN J 2002;75(6):1143–58.
7. Ethicon Endo-Surgery, I. (2007). Looking beneath the surface: the facts about reprocessing single-use devices.
8. FDA shares data on events related to the reuse of singe-use devices. OR Manager 2006;22(11):1–5.
9. Association of Operating Room Nurses. Perioperative standards and recommended practices. AORN guidance statement: reuse of single-use devices. Denver (CO): AORN; 2010. p. 649–55.

Future Trends in Sterilization and Disinfection

Pamela Carter, RN, BSN, CNOR*, M. Chris King, RN, CRCST,
Linda Clement, BSM, CRCST

KEYWORDS

• Sterilization • Disinfection • Chemical indicators • Aldehyde

In the operating room (OR), patient outcomes are highly sensitive to the quality of clinical practice; perioperative nursing practice has a significant impact on patient safety. The OR, like the cockpit of an airplane, is a place where being methodical and meticulous and following an established routine is highly effective. In such a controlled environment, changing practice is not easy. Considering changing a practice that has promoted good patient outcomes for a new way of doing things can be uncomfortable and can meet with resistance.

The more impact a practice has on patient safety, the harder it is to change. For example, the transition from determining the sterility of instruments with an expiration date to accepting that an item remains sterile until something happens to contaminate it (event-related sterility) was a very slow process. Sterile instruments are essential to patient safety. Even though event-related sterility saves a significant amount of money in labor and supplies, the old practice had proven results. The more important the outcome of a process, the harder it is to contemplate changing it, even to save time or money; if the new approach does not work, the consequences could be devastating.

Perioperative nurses should keep abreast of the new technologies that are being developed. A new technology can represent a significant advance in the ability to achieve good patient outcomes. New technologies can also represent opportunities to improve efficiency and reduce the cost of health care. Improvements on current technology are readily incorporated into practice, but a new technology, which challenges a tried and true practice, can take much longer to adopt.

STERIS Corporation, 5960 Heisley Road, Mentor, OH 44060, USA
* Corresponding author.
E-mail address: Pamela_Carter@steris.com

Perioperative Nursing Clinics 5 (2010) 383–391
doi:10.1016/j.cpen.2010.05.001   **periopnursing.theclinics.com**

CLASS 6 EMULATING INDICATORS AND OXIDATIVE HIGH-LEVEL DISINFECTION
Class 6 Emulating Indicators: A Future Trend that is Already Here

Steam sterilization has been used in health care for more than 100 years, and it is still the safest, most cost effective, and easily understood method to sterilize critical items that can withstand high temperature and moisture.[1] The principles of steam sterilization have not changed over the years, but the way the process is monitored is evolving. Perioperative professionals should be aware of the latest sterilization monitoring technologies and their significance, because these products can directly impact the perioperative environment.

The Introduction of Chemical Indicators for Health Care Processes

In the late 1940s and early 1950s, chemical indicators (CIs) were introduced to monitor the steam sterilization process.[2] The first CIs used simplistic chemical reactions that occurred when the indicator was presented with sterilization conditions. These simple throughput indicators provided little information about the sterilization process, but were able to detect certain procedural failures. However, as with many other medical practices and devices, advancements in the understanding of the sterilization process have led to advancements in CIs. Today's indicators use complex chemical reactions and provide significantly more information about the steam sterilization process.

Current Classifications

There were no classifications for CIs until December 1988, when the Association for the Advancement of Medical Instrumentation (AAMI) published a technical report titled "The Selection and Use of CIs for Steam Sterilization Monitoring in Health Care Facilities.[1]"

CIs are defined by AAMI as "...sterilization process monitoring devices designed to respond with a chemical or physical change to one or more of the physical conditions within the sterilizing chamber. CIs assist in the detection of potential sterilization failures that could result from incorrect packaging, incorrect loading of the sterilizer, or malfunctions of the sterilizer.[3]"

Today, American National Standards Institute (ANSI)/AAMI/International Organization for Standardization (ISO) 11140-1:2005 defines 6 classes of CIs and specifies performance requirements for each of them:

1. Process indicators (Class 1): These CIs are used to indicate that an item has been exposed to the sterilization process and used to distinguish between processed and unprocessed items; they are referred to as external CIs.[4] Examples of Class 1 indicators are instrument tape and the external indicators found on peel pouches.
2. Indicators for use in specific tests (Class 2): These indicators are also known as specialty indicators, and are designed for use in specific test procedures as defined by sterilization standards.[4] An example of Class 2 indicators is the Bowie-Dick (air removal) test. This indicator tests for the presence of air in the sterilizer chamber, and a positive test would mean that air, which inhibits steam from contacting all surfaces of an item, has either not been removed during the cycle or has entered the chamber through leaks in the system.
3. Single-parameter indicators (Class 3): These indicators are designed to react to one of the critical parameters of steam sterilization and to indicate exposure to a sterilization cycle at stated values of the chosen parameters.[4] The critical parameters usually chosen are time or temperature.
4. Multiparameter indicators (Class 4): These indicators are designed to react to 2 or more of the critical parameters of sterilization and to indicate exposure to the cycle

at stated values of the chosen parameters. Time and temperature are the typical steam sterilization parameters used.[4] The Class 4 indicators are more accurate than Class 3 indicators.

5. Integrating indicators (Class 5): These indicators, which are also known as integrators, react to all the critical parameters over a specified range of sterilization cycles, and their performance has been correlated to the performance of a biologic indicator (BI) under the labeled conditions for use.[4]

6. Class 6 emulating indicators are also known as cycle-specific indicators. Each indicator must demonstrate that it meets all the critical parameters of sterilization for a specific sterilization cycle. Each Class 6 indicator is made to monitor the specific temperature and time of a chosen steam sterilization cycle. If the Class 6 indicator is included inside a test pack, the test pack would also be specific to the preconditioning process of a cycle, such as dynamic air removal (vacuum-assisted) or gravity displacement test packs. This factor is what makes these cycle-specific indicators different from the Class 5 integrating indicators.

Class 6 is New to the United States

Class 6 emulating indicators are the latest addition to the ANSI/AAMI standards.[4] However, this technology has been used in other parts of the world for many years. The technology was first adopted by AAMI in 2005 as part of the global harmonization of the CI performance document ST60 to the new global document ANSI/AAMI/ISO 11140-1. This adoption defined performance criteria and expectations for a new category of CIs, Class 6 emulating indicators. Although ANSI/AAMI/ISO 11140-1 incorporated Class 6 emulating indicators, no recommended practices were assigned or adopted. Class 6 emulating indicators were not sold in the United States at that time. Without Food and Drug Administration (FDA) clearance for a product being used by hospital facilities, guidelines could not be developed. In fact, the discussion of Class 6 in the ANSI/AAMI/ISO 11140-1 document was only done to facilitate global acceptance of the document.

How and Why is it Different?

The Class 5 integrating indicator is designed to mimic the performance of a BI.[3] In the case of steam sterilization, it would mimic the performance of a BI for a specific temperature range. However, the integrating indicator does not draw a distinction among exposure times for a given temperature. Even though one steam sterilization temperature setting (eg, 270°F/132°C) may be used for multiple cycles with varying exposure times (3-minute flash, 4-minute prevacuum, 10-minute flash, 15-minute gravity), the 270°F integrating indicator is designed to show a passing result at the same point that a BI dies, which correlates to the shortest exposure time for that temperature. In this example, the Class 5 integrating indicator is designed to pass after exposure to 3 minutes of steam at 270°F; this means that regardless of the 270°F cycle chosen, it only monitors the 3-minute time.

In contrast, when using Class 6 emulating indicators, staff would choose the specific indicator designed for each exposure time.[5,6] The ink would display the pass color change on reaching the 3-minute, 4-minute, 10-minute, or 15-minute exposure time for that particular cycle.

Tight Performance Requirements

A Class 6 emulating indicator must also meet tight specifications for performance. **Table 1** shows the performance specifications identified in ANSI/AAMI/ISO 11140-1.[4] These specifications indicate that a Class 6 emulating indicator shows passing

Table 1
Performance requirements of Class 6 emulating steam indicators as identified by ANSI/AAMI/ISO 11140-1

Test Point	Test Time	Test Temperature	Test Condition
Steam passing condition	SV	SV	Saturated steam
Steam failing condition	SV 6%	SV – 1°C	Saturated steam
Dry heat test (indicator must fail)	30 min	137°C	Dry heat

Abbreviation: SV, stated value: selected based on the critical variable required for a specified sterilization cycle.

conditions at the stated value, such as 4 minutes of exposure to saturated steam at 132°C (270°F), for example, but show failing conditions when exposed to 94% of the exposure time and 1°C lower temperature.[4] In this example, the failing condition would be 131°C (268°F) for 3.76 minutes. **Table 2** gives the exposure conditions of common sterilization cycles and the pass or fail expectations for Class 6 emulating indicators used for those cycles.

What this all Means for the Perioperative Department

In a sterile processing department, indicators and challenge packs are used in conjunction with biologic monitoring of the sterilizers, physical monitors, accurate record keeping, and a sterilizer preventive maintenance program.[1,3,7] Because the Class 6 emulating indicators offer a means to monitor all the specific requirements of a particular sterilization cycle, Class 6 challenge packs allow the sterile processing staff to release sterilized loads quickly after processing and cooling, which helps speed up delivery of instruments to the perioperative department.[8–10]

In the OR, staff must confirm the sterility of the items coming from a sterile processing department to make sure they are safe to use for surgery and diagnostic procedures.[7] There are 3 checkpoints for OR staff to complete:

1. Inspect the external integrity of packages, trays, and containers for any rips, holes, or major dents. If the integrity of the device is compromised, it must be reprocessed.

Table 2
Typical steam sterilization cycles and the performance expectations of Class 6 emulating indicators

Steam Sterilization Cycle Parameters[3]	Class 6 Emulating Ink-Stated Values	Steam Pass Conditions	Steam Fail Conditions
30-min gravity cycle at 250°F/ 121°C[4]	121°C 30 min	121°C 30 min	120°C 28.2 min
3-min gravity flash sterilization cycle at 270°F/132°C	132°C 3 min	132°C 3 min	131°C 2.82 min
10-min gravity flash sterilization cycle at 270°F/132°C	132°C 10 min	132°C 10 min	131°C 9.4 min
4-min prevacuum sterilization cycle at 270°F/132°C	132°C 4 min	132°C 4 min	131°C 3.76 min
15-min gravity sterilization cycle at 270°F/132°C	132°C 15 min	132°C 15 min	131°C 14.1 min
3-minute prevacuum sterilization cycle at 275°F/135°C	135°C 3 min	135°C 3 min	134°C 2.82 min

2. Check the Class 1 indicator (instrument tape, indicator card) on the outside of the item to make sure it has been through a sterilization process.
3. Verify that the CI inside each package, tray, or container has also passed.

It is important for perioperative staff to remember that a passing CI does not assure that the items are sterile; it indicates that the parameters for sterilization, which the CI was designed to measure, have been met.[1,7] The sterile processing staff is responsible for making sure that all of the other measures of sterility have been met before they send any items to the OR for use.[11]

Flashing in the Surgical Suite

Flash sterilization should be kept to a minimum and used in limited clinical situations in a controlled manner.[7] It is not a substitute for purchasing sufficient instrument inventory. If flash sterilization is being performed in the OR, then everyone who sterilizes in the department is responsible for making sure that all measures of steam sterilization are met. Staff must perform regular biologic testing of the sterilizers, use physical monitors, use internal CIs in every load, and maintain accurate and complete records of cycles run in the department.[7] It is important that for optimal sterility assurance, the CI should be placed in areas least accessible to steam penetration.[3,6] This location may or may not be at the center of the package, tray, or container system.

Until recently, only Classes 3, 4, and 5 CIs were available for monitoring flashed loads. However, if a surgical implant was flashed, AAMI and AORN standards and guidelines required that the load contain a CI and a BI. These guidelines also required that the items in the flashed load be quarantined until the results of the BI were known.[7] In actual practice, there are times when the processed implantable device is used before knowing the results of the BI, but this practice should not be promoted.

New Option for Monitoring Flash Cycles: Extended Cycles

Using Class 6 technology in flash loads gives perioperative staff immediate results and greater assurance that the sterilizer achieved all of the critical steam sterilization parameters (time, temperature, and saturation/quality of steam). It also assures staff that the indicator's pass is correlated to the specific cycle that was run, within a tighter tolerance range, so the items can be released immediately.[8–10]

The Class 6 emulating indicator strips and challenge packs also provide a sterility assurance monitoring solution for one of the medical device industry's more recent sterility assurance challenges; extended cycles.

Medical devices and instrument sets have become more complex over time, providing a greater challenge to air removal and steam penetration. These devices and sets require longer exposure times to achieve sterilization. Earlier sterility assurance indicators were not designed or cleared by the FDA for monitoring these extended cycles. Because the Class 6 emulating indicators are cycle-specific and are available for longer cycle times, they provide the sterilization monitoring solution for these extended cycles.

Class 6 emulating indicators and challenge packs have been cleared to monitor the extended cycle times listed in the new AAMI TIR31, process challenge devices, or test packs for use in health care facilities. These times include the 270°F, 10-minute prevacuum steam sterilization cycle and the 270°F, 20-minute prevacuum steam sterilization cycle.

New Product Awaits Guidance

Guidance groups such as AAMI, AORN, and Centers for Disease Control and Prevention have not yet established policies for use of the Class 6 emulating indicators. CI strips and CI challenge packs are being marketed in the United States and around the world today. The various manufacturers' instructions indicate that these products are intended to be used to monitor the internal confines of pouches, trays, and rigid sterilization containers, and indicate that the challenge packs may be used to monitor all loads.[8–10]

AORN and AAMI clearly state in their published guidance that as new medical devices and technologies are cleared by the FDA, facilities should activate a multidisciplinary action team that comprises knowledgable experts to select the best monitoring devices for the hospital.[3,7] Areas of expertise should include, but are not limited to, surgical services, sterile processing, infection control, and administration. Facilities should review the instructions provided with the product, confirm clearance by FDA, obtain testing data provided by manufacturers, and perform a product evaluation appropriate for the product's intended application in the facility. The optimal products should be selected based on evidence-based scientific data and product performance characteristics, and not on personal preference or because of a fear of change.[3,7]

Class 6 emulating indicators seem to be here to stay. These indicators are gaining popularity for use in the perioperative suite and in sterile processing departments, because there is factual evidence of their clinical performance. Class 6 emulating indicators are cost-competitive, compatible with the most current practices, and easy to use; they are generally reliable and monitor more of the steam sterilization cycle, which provides a greater safety margin.[8–10] Even more, they offer perioperative and sterile processing teams the opportunity to improve efficiency in the OR and the sterile processing department. It is only a matter of time before guidance is forthcoming to encourage best practices for the use of Class 6 technology.

NEW OXIDATIVE MULTIPURPOSE LIQUID HIGH-LEVEL DISINFECTANT: A SIGNIFICANT ADVANCE FOR ENDOSCOPES

Surgical and endoscopy staff has been using high-level disinfectants to process heat-sensitive medical devices for many years. These chemistries are used to process scopes between patient uses and render them safe for use in noninvasive procedures. However, some older disinfection chemistries have caused some problems for patients, staff, devices, and even the environment.

Some of the early aldehyde-based products were associated with respiratory irritation from the strong fumes emitted from the solution when staff was working with them. In addition, if all contaminants were not removed from medical devices (and particularly the insides of flexible endoscope lumens) during cleaning, the binding properties of aldehyde-based products would help to affix debris to the device surfaces, which could later break free.[12] This problem could occur during a subsequent cleaning or potentially during a patient procedure. There has also been the potential for patients to develop dialdehyde-induced colitis, and some patient deaths have even been linked to improper rinsing of processed devices before reuse.[13,14] Some high-level disinfectants also require special ventilation and pose a toxicity hazard to the environment. Therefore, these disinfectants require neutralizing before disposal.

Oxidative chemistries and processing systems have been gaining popularity in sterile processing departments and surgical centers for reprocessing heat-sensitive surgical instruments, because oxidative chemistries and processing systems are considered to be safe and nonstaining when used according to manufacturers' directions. However, they have only recently been applied to high-level disinfection processes.

A New Oxidative Problem Solver

Although progress in developing faster and safer high-level disinfectants has been painfully slow, improvements have finally been achieved that eliminate the primary concerns related to previous chemistries. A new high-level disinfection solution has been developed that offers solutions to existing patient, staff, device, and environmental issues. This formula was previously available in Canada and elsewhere and is now available in the United States.

This new oxidative chemistry is a broad-based microbicide made from a proprietary formulation that combines a low 2% concentration of hydrogen peroxide (H_2O_2) with other inert ingredients to provide accelerated efficacy. This new oxidative has a very mild odor, is free rinsing and highly effective, and is environmentally friendly.

How Does it Work?

Oxidative compounds contain an additional atom of oxygen. These products use oxidation to interrupt cellular functions that kills the microorganisms. The mechanism of action is nonspecific, but it has to do with the loss of molecular structure and function. Oxidating products also exhibit excellent cleaning, disinfecting, and sterilizing properties. Milder versions of this type of compound can be found for household use ("Oxy" products and H_2O_2 solution used for cuts and infections).

Because this new formulation only requires a single rinse (compared with older chemistries that require 2–3 rinses), overall processing times may be reduced by 5 to 10 minutes in both manual soaking processes and in automated endoscope processors (AERs). With such a low concentration of H_2O_2, this new high-level disinfectant offers excellent material compatibility and can be reused for up to 21 days. The ready-to-use, high-level disinfectant was designed to be used in a facility's existing AERs.

A Culture Shift

This oxidative disinfection option is a significant advance forward, but it requires an adjustment for the endoscopy department. Change is always a challenge, but a change for the better is worth the effort. This change does not require reinventing the wheel; a facility's current disinfection protocols and procedures can still be used, but can be pared down somewhat. For example, steps involving neutralizing a solution before disposal are no longer needed. Members of staff appreciate the benefits of a faster, easier, and safer process once they see the difference for themselves.

HYDROGEN PEROXIDE STERILIZATION

H_2O_2 is a naturally occurring water-like liquid that has impressive antimicrobial and disinfectant properties, effectively killing bacteria, viruses, and fungi. Since 1905, it has been used in low concentration (3%) as a household disinfectant and to disinfect skin abrasions and lesions. In higher concentrations (50%–90%), H_2O_2 has long been used as a sterilant in the pharmaceutical industry, and in aerospace research it is used to sterilize satellites. H_2O_2 is also less hazardous to employees than other low-temperature sterilants; its by-products, water and oxygen, are safe for the environment.

Gaseous H_2O_2 sterilization is rapidly becoming the technology of choice for items that are heat- and moisture-sensitive, and is replacing ethylene oxide (EtO). H_2O_2 sterilization is cost effective, reliable, and safe. Compared with EtO, the capital investment and operational costs of H_2O_2 sterilizers are lower, the sterilization process is significantly shorter, there are no safety issues involved for employees and patients, and items can be used immediately following sterilization (no aeration or drying time is required).

The first H_2O_2 sterilizer for the surgical market was introduced in 1993 using a technology that creates a gas plasma with the H_2O_2 as part of its sterilization process. Gas plasma is not required for H_2O_2 sterilization, and more recently vaporized H_2O_2 sterilizers that do not use plasma have been introduced in the surgical setting.

There are material restrictions with all H_2O_2 sterilization technologies: liquids, linens, powders, and cellulose are incompatible with H_2O_2. There are also lumen restrictions associated with H_2O_2 sterilization. However, the specific items that can or cannot be sterilized in a particular sterilizer are determined not necessarily by the sterilization technology but by what the manufacturer validated and submitted in the 510(k) that was cleared by the FDA.

In machines of the same size, the chamber in a vaporized H_2O_2 sterilizer can be more productively used than an H_2O_2 plasma sterilizer chamber, because it does not have to accommodate a plasma coil. Good practice dictates that items processed in a sterilizer should not contact the walls of the chamber. However, load shift sometimes occurs, leading to sterilization cycle aborts in H_2O_2 plasma sterilization. Residual moisture, even on instruments that have been properly cleaned and dried, can cause an aborted cycle in a H_2O_2 plasma. Vaporized H_2O_2 is less sensitive to residual moisture. Aborted sterilization cycles can be costly in terms of the time that items are out of service and the time and supplies required to repackage the items for resterilization.

Some H_2O_2 sterilizers have dual cycles, one for lumened items that take more time to sterilize and a shorter cycle for nonlumened items. This option increases efficiency, because the user can choose the shorter cycle time when no lumens are included in the load.

With the increase in complex surgical devices and instrumentation that are heat- and moisture-sensitive, hospitals are becoming more and more dependent on low-temperature sterilization. The rapid cycle times and sterile storage capability of H_2O_2 sterilization combined with its safety ensure that the utility of this sterilization method and its use in the surgical setting will only increase.

SUMMARY

It is important for the perioperative team to stay abreast of new trends in health care, especially those that may directly affect their patients and departments. In the case of steam sterilization, Class 6 emulating indicators are so new that guidance is not yet available for their use. However, as increasing numbers of health care facilities implement their own best practices for monitoring programs and protocols that incorporate Class 6 technology, standards will evolve to include them.

In departments that reprocess endoscopes and other temperature-sensitive devices, there is a new, ready-to-use oxidative high-level disinfectant available for use in the United States. Once perioperative professionals understand the significant potential benefits to patients, department staff, and their expensive devices, changing from an aldehyde-based formulation to an oxidative one would be a sensible option.

With the rapid increase in complex heat- and moisture-sensitive surgical instrumentation, cost effective, safe, and efficient sterilants such as H_2O_2 become increasingly valuable. Facilities determine their sterilization choices based on how a particular sterilization technology and brand of sterilizer meets their space requirements, cost constraints, types and quantities of instruments they have in inventory, and their need to control instrument turnover between procedures, among other factors.

REFERENCES

1. Reichert M, Young J. Sterilization technology for the health care facility. 2nd edition. Gaithersburg (MD): Aspen Publications; 1997.
2. Kurowski J. Chemical indicators 101: application for use. Infection Control Today Nov 2004.
3. Comprehensive guide to steam sterilization and sterility assurance in health care facilities; Association for the Advancement of Medical Instrumentation. Arlington (VA): ANSI/AAMI ST79;2006 (A1:2008, A2:2009).
4. Sterilization of health care products—chemical indicators—part 1; general requirements. Association for the Advancement of Medical Instrumentation. Arlington (VA): ANSI/AAMI/ISO 11140:1;2005.
5. Sterilization of health care products chemical indicators-guidance for the selection, use and interpretation of results. Association for the Advancement of Medical Instrumentation. Arlington (VA): ANSI/AAMI/ISO 15882; 2008.
6. Spry C. Understanding current steam sterilization recommendations and guidelines. AORN J 2008;88(4):537–54.
7. Standards recommended practices and guidelines; recommended practices for sterilization in the perioperative practice setting. Arlington (VA): Association of Perioperative Registered Nurses (AORN); 2009.
8. Gray E. Sterile processing quality improvement at CoxHealth. Healthcare Purchasing News March 2009.
9. Blasko R. Class 6 vs. BIs: can't we all just get along? Infection Control Today August 2009.
10. Clement L, Ames H, Carter P, et al. Reduce flash sterilization errors, eliminate blind release and increase sterilization productivity. STERIS Corporation White Paper September 2008.
11. Central service technical manual. 7th edition. Chicago (IL): IAHCSMM (International Association of Healthcare Central Service Materiel Management); 2007.
12. McDonnell GE. Antisepsis, disinfection, and sterilization: types, action, and resistance. Washington, DC: ASM Press; 2007.
13. West AB, Kuan SF, Bennick M, et al. Glutaraldehyde colitis following endoscopy: clinical and pathological features and investigation of an outbreak, case report. Gastroenterology 1995. Elsevier BV.
14. Stein BL, Lamoureux E, Miller M. Glutaraldehyde-induced colitis. Can J Surg 2001. Available at: www.ncbi.nlm.nih.gov/pubmed/11308232. Accessed September 1, 2009.

Effective Management of Loaner Instrumentation

Nancy Chobin, RN, AAS, ACSP, CSPDM

KEYWORDS

- Loaner instrumentation • Perioperative nurse
- Patient safety • Cost containment

The increasing sophistication of surgical procedures that requires special instrumentation has made the management of loaner instrumentation a major responsibility for perioperative nurses in assuring patient safety.[1–6] Cost containment initiatives have increased facilities' dependence on loaner instruments as they reduce the need to purchase seldom-used specialty instrumentation, which often relates only to a specific procedure. In reality, it is virtually impossible for any facility to purchase all the instrumentation required for every specialty case, making the need for loaner instrumentation vital to patient care.

Although loaner instrumentation can include sets borrowed from another health care facility or physician-owned instrumentation that is brought in for specific cases, most often loaner instrumentation is obtained from a variety of vendors. Much of this instrumentation is specifically designed for implants that can be used only in conjunction with the borrowed instruments.

The implications for management of loaner instrumentation are the same as for inpatient and ambulatory surgery facilities. To insure patient safety, avoid costly delays in the operating room, and facilitate surgeon satisfaction, it is essential that a comprehensive policy and procedure for the management of loaner instruments be developed, in-serviced, implemented, and monitored for compliance.

POLICY CONSIDERATIONS

Effective management of loaner instrumentation requires a collaborative effort among several departments, including, at minimum, perioperative services (including surgeon input), sterile processing department (SPD) or central service department, infection control, purchasing, materials management, and receiving. A vendor is one of the most important partners in effective loaner management. Vendors must understand a facility's requirements for ordering, receiving, and returning loaner instrumentation, including who is accountable at each stage in the process.

Saint Barnabas Healthcare System, West Orange, NJ, USA
E-mail address: nancy.chobin@att.net

Perioperative Nursing Clinics 5 (2010) 393–396
doi:10.1016/j.cpen.2010.04.003
1556-7931/10/$ – see front matter © 2010 Elsevier Inc. All rights reserved.
periopnursing.theclinics.com

INSTRUCTIONS FOR USE

Borrowed instruments may require special cleaning agents, implements, and protocols that differ from what are used for a facility's basic instruments. A device or instrument set's design, construction, or material can provide unique challenges to effective cleaning or sterilization. Looks can be deceiving. A perioperative nurse should never assume that specialty instruments can be cleaned and or sterilized "as usual." Facilities should require that all loaner devices and instrumentation be accompanied by manufacturer instructions. For instance, the type and pH of cleaning agent may be significant, and some devices can be adversely affected by high pH detergents. Vendors should provide a count sheet with each set's contents, including the name of each instrument, its catalog number, and how many of each instrument are in the set (**Box 1**).

WEIGHT OF SETS AND CONTAINERS

The Association for the Advancement of Medical Instrumentation's "Containment Devices for Reusable Medical Device Sterilization," recommends a maximum weight for loaner sets of 25 pounds, which includes the weight of the container. Sets weighing more than 25 pounds present ergonomic issues for operating room (OR) and SPD personnel. In addition, heavier sets and certain container materials make drying instruments properly more difficult. Facilities should weigh loaner sets for compliance with this standard. Vendors can repackage heavier sets into more than one container.

TIME LINE

Facilities should specify how far in advance of scheduled cases of loaner instruments must arrive. This requires that facilities know the turnaround time specific to each loaner device or instrument set. Extended cleaning or sterilization protocols required for an instrument or device must be factored into the turnaround time calculation. This advance time requirement should be part of a facility's loaner policy. In addition, a policy should

---

Box 1
A manufacturer's recommended cleaning protocol should include at a minimum

- Soak time (eg, in an enzymatic detergent)
- Use of ultrasonic cleaner and length of cleaning cycle
- Use of mechanical cleaner (eg, washer-decontaminator)
- Use of instrument lubricant (some manufacturers of metal implants do not recommend the use of lubricants on the metal screws or plates)
- Assembly instructions (eg, any items that must be disassembled for sterilization)
- Specific sterilization instructions, including
  - Sterilization methodology
  - Cycle type (eg, gravity displacement or dynamic air removal cycle)
  - Exposure temperature
  - Exposure time (may be different for sets with instruments only vs sets containing implants)
  - Dry time recommended (this is usually a minimal time; facilities should use a dry time that produces dry sets at the completion of the cycle)

specify what action is taken if a vendor fails to comply (eg, the surgeon is notified that the procedure must be rescheduled to accommodate the required preparation time).

COMMUNICATIONS

The availability of loaner information for scheduled cases requires adequate staffing in the processing department, especially if several loaner sets are scheduled for a single procedure or if loaner sets are needed for different procedures at the same time. A comprehensive communication tool can insure that everyone involved in readying a loaner set for use is apprised of the information needed. The communication tool should contain, at minimum, surgeon name and procedure, date and time of sched-uled surgery, number of sets required for the procedure, how and when the sets will arrive, and any special instructions that differ from routine instrument processing protocols that might require additional preparation time.

RECORD KEEPING

Accountability for loaner instruments is essential. Sterile processing should maintain records, including when the instruments were received, time received, name of the person checking in the loaner sets, the sets used, copies of manufacturers' instructions for use, if all the items were present and in working order (requires a count sheet) when the sets arrived, name of person checking out the instruments (back to the vendor), and when they were returned. In addition, any items damaged (on receipt or during use) should be documented. Many facilities use a form to track instruments throughout the process; others use computerized surgical instrument tracking systems.

ORDERING PROTOCOLS

A policy should delineate how the loaner instruments are ordered, who is responsible for this task, and where the loaner instruments should be delivered (eg, SPD or decon-tamination area).

RETURN PROTOCOLS

A policy should delineate how loaner sets are processed before they are returned to the vendor. It is essential that loaner instruments be cleaned according to manufac-turers' instructions before and after use. It is inexcusable for loaner instruments to be returned improperly cleaned. Some vendors charge facilities a cleaning fee if loaner instruments are returned improperly cleaned. There must be a mechanism in place to verify that all instruments are accounted for and in working order.

A specific individual (or position title) should be identified to whom reprocessed loaner sets must be delivered for return to the vendor. This individual should record the date and time of receipt of the instruments, identify the appropriate purchase order number, and obtain the signature of the person delivering the instruments. A policy should define how the loaner items will be returned (eg, courier) and who makes the arrangements for the return. If loaner sets are picked up, designate a time frame (eg, within 48 hours of the surgery); loaner sets can take up a great deal of space. If an individual picks up a set, the records should include the time, date, and name and signature of that person. A facility should be held responsible for items lost or damaged during the time the instruments were in the facility. If patient charges are applicable, these charges should be verified.

PROCESSING STAFF TRAINING AND COMPETENCY ASSESSMENTS

With the wide variation in loaner set configurations and the cleaning challenges associated with many of these sets, it is critical that all staff responsible for loaner instruments be thoroughly trained and knowledgeable of the loaner policy as well as manufacturers' recommended processing protocols. In-servicing must be provided for staff competency verification and documentation. Adherence to an effective protocol prevents just-in-time delivery of loaner instrumentation that keeps staff from being properly in-serviced.

DAMAGED/SOILED INSTRUMENTS

Loaner policies should address what actions to take if instruments arrive damaged. Document problems (damaged instruments should be documented and reported to the vendor). Loaner sets require wrapping; few vendors provide sets in a container that does not require additional packaging. Therefore, preventing damage to sets is important to prevent delays in an OR (including the need to flash sterilize). SPD and the OR should collaboratively develop preventive measures to protect trays from damage, including placing trays on a separate covered or enclosed cart, use of plastic protective transfer trays (provided by the packaging manufacturer), and not permitting stacking of loaner sets.

MONITORING OF PROCESSES

All of a policy's considerations should be monitored for compliance. This is especially true for cleaning and sterilization protocols.

SUMMARY

Effective management of loaner instruments, including a clearly written policy, is essential for patient safety, cost containment, and surgeon satisfaction. Quality issues (such as improperly cleaned, missing, or damaged instruments) can cause delays in patient care and potential never events in surgical patients. Delays in an OR due to instrumentation issues result in lost revenue to the facility. Accountability for loaner instrumentation can prevent costly delays and expenses related to missing or damaged items, including those that did not occur at a borrower's facility.

REFERENCES

1. ANSI/AAMI ST-79:2006, Annex II. Comprehensive guide to steam sterilization and sterility assurance in health care facilities. Arlington (VA), 2009.
2. Association of PeriOperative Registered Nurses. Recommended practices for sterilization in the perioperative practice setting. Denver (CO), March 2009.
3. Association of PeriOperative Registered Nurses. Recommended practices for cleaning and care ofg surgical instruments and powered equipment. Denver (CO), March 2009.
4. Chobin N, Evans C, Japp N, et al. Roles and responsibilities. In: Chobin N, editor. The basics of sterile processing. 2nd edition. Kenilworth (NJ): Backer Printing, Inc; 2008. Chapters 5 and 7.
5. Chobin N. Management basics for sterile processing. 1st edition. Kenilworth (NJ): Backer Printing; 2008.
6. Huter-Kunish G. Processing loaner instruments in an ambulatory surgery center. AORN J 2009;89(5).

TASS Prevention for Perioperative Nurses

Susan Clouser, RN, MSN, CRNO

KEYWORDS

- TASS • Endophthalmitis • Toxic anterior segment syndrome
- Perioperative

One might be surprised to find an article on toxic anterior segment syndrome (TASS) in a text dedicated to disinfection and sterilization, two processes critical to preventing postoperative infections, because TASS is not an infection.

TASS is an acute, sterile inflammation of the anterior chamber of the eye after an intraocular procedure, most often cataract surgery. It occurs when a noninfectious substance enters the eye during or after a surgical procedure that results in intraocular inflammation.

When sterility is compromised and a true bacterial infection of the eye occurs, it is termed, *endophthalmitis*. According to medical terminology, endophthalmitis (meaning inside, the eye, and inflammation) could also describe TASS. The diagnosis of endophthalmitis, however, has always implied a bacterial origin.

If a patient has postoperative inflammation and the intraocular fluids are tapped and cultured in an attempt to determine the most effective antibiotic for treatment and the culture is negative, it is said that the patient has sterile endophthalmitis. This term is a misnomer because it implies inflammation in all chambers of the globe rather than in the anterior segment. The more accurate term, *toxic anterior segment syndrome,* was coined by Monson and colleagues[1] in 1992.

Although TASS is not caused by bacteria, except indirectly in the case of endotoxin, its signs and symptoms are similar to endophthalmitis. They include decreased visual acuity, increased cell and flare (indicators of anterior chamber inflammation), and, often, limbus-to-limbus corneal edema. In severe cases, there may be fibrin in the anterior chamber and a hypopyon (pus in the eye) may be present.

Because the symptoms of TASS are similar to endophthalmitis, the diagnosis is often missed. A key factor in differentiating between the two is the time frame during which the inflammation develops. Classic endophthalmitis takes 48 to 72 hours to become symptomatic whereas TASS becomes evident in the first 24 hours post surgery. Differentiation is critical because the treatments are different and the treatment for one is not appropriate for the other.

640 Post Oak Drive, Plano, TX 75025, USA
E-mail address: eyenursetx@verizon.net

Perioperative Nursing Clinics 5 (2010) 397–399
doi:10.1016/j.cpen.2010.04.004   **periopnursing.theclinics.com**

The key to preventing TASS from occurring in an operating room is in understanding the potential causes and eliminating them from your practice. The most important preventative measure in the war against TASS is proper instrument cleaning. An ad hoc task force was convened in September 2006 by the American Society of Cataract and Refractive Surgery and the American Society of Ophthalmic Registered Nurses to determine appropriate methods for cleaning eye instruments. The task force consisted of doctors, nurses, and representatives from industry, the Food and Drug Administration, and the Centers for Disease Control. The work of this committee produced the document *Recommended Practices for Cleaning and Sterilizing Intraocular Surgical Instruments*,[2] published in 2007.

The following key points are made in these recommended practices:

All debris and ophthalmic viscosurgical devices (OVDs) must be removed from instrumentation by manual cleaning. Keeping instruments moist until cleaning begins makes the process easier.

Follow the manufacturer's directions for use (DFUs) when cleaning any piece of equipment, in particular phacoemulsification hand pieces and irrigation/aspiration tips and hand pieces.

Use instrument-cleaning detergents and enzymatic cleaners according to manufacturers' DFUs. Assure that all instruments are thoroughly rinsed to ensure removal of all detergents and cleaners.

Use disposable cannulas and tubing whenever possible and do not reuse single use devices.

If an ultrasonic cleaner is used it should be dedicated to ophthalmic instruments. The water should be changed frequently and the unit should be drained and cleaned at the end of the day to prevent endotoxin.

Instruments should be sterilized according to manufacturers' DFUs.

Particulate matter on the intraocular lens (IOL) follows instrument cleaning as a leading cause of TASS. The IOL should never come in contact with anything but the package it comes in, balanced salt irrigating solution or OVD to lubricate it, the forceps used to pick it up, and the cartridge it is inserted in for implantation.

The lens should not be placed on a glove or other surface to change or correct the grip nor should the lens be touched with a gloved finger to manipulate its placement in the insertion cartridge. Surgical gloves are sterile, but sterility is not the issue, toxicity is. By the time the lens is introduced to the sterile field, the gloves of the scrub person have been in contact with multiple items, including lint-producing items, such as towels and 4 × 4 gauze sponges. In addition, when gloves are manufactured, a releasing compound is used on the glove mold to aid in the gloves' removal. Some of the compound remains on the glove and can be transferred to the IOL.

Finally it is important to assure that all medications used inside the eye or immediately postoperatively contain no preservatives. Preoperative medications, such as dilating drops, are normally not a problem because they are rinsed away by the tears before the incision. What can be an issue are medications that are viscous or gel-like in nature, especially if they contain preservatives. If these substances are instilled in the cul-de-sac before surgery, it is possible that some may remain and be carried into the anterior chamber on an instrument. Thorough irrigation of the cul-de-sac during the surgical prep or after insertion of the speculum helps remove these medications.

Often a surgeon requests that epinephrine or antibiotics be added to the irrigating solution used with the phacoemulsification machine. If preserved medications are used for this purpose, they are introduced to the inside of the eye during the phacoemulsification and irrigation and aspiration portions of the procedure. Manufacturers recommend that the products be used as delivered, without additives. Adding anything to an irrigating solution makes the facility the "manufacturer of the product" and voids a manufacturer's warranty.

Any medication delivered directly to the anterior chamber, such as lidocaine, epinephrine, or a combination of these, used to promote dilation should also be preservative-free.

In the same way, eyedrops instilled postoperatively should be preservative-free. Eyedrops and ointment[3] are capable of entering the eye through a clear corneal incision that is not completely sealed and may lead to TASS. For the same reason, povidone iodine should not be instilled in the cul-de-sac postoperatively.

There are many possible causes of TASS, but the majority of cases result from inadequate instrument cleaning, transfer of particulate matter, especially on the IOL, and preservatives in medications. Paying strict attention to these key areas prevents TASS in most cases.

REFERENCES

1. Monson MC, Mamalis N, Olson RJ. Toxic anterior segment inflammation following cataract surgery. J Cataract Refract Surg 1992;18:184–9.
2. Hellinger WC, Bacalis LP, Edelhauser HF, et al. Recommended practices for cleaning and sterilizing intraocular surgical instruments. J Cataract Refract Surg 2007; 33:1095–100.
3. Werner L, Sher JH, Taylor JR, et al. Toxic anterior segment syndrome and possible association with ointment in the anterior chamber following cataract surgery. J Cataract Refract Surg 2006;32:227–35.

Index

Note: Page numbers of article titles are in **boldface** type.

A

Accountability, in infection prevention, 356
Advocacy, for infection prevention, 356–367
Agency for Healthcare Administration, inspections by, 348–351
ALPHA patrols, **347–353**
American Society for Gastrointestinal Endoscopy, equipment reprocessing
    recommendations of, 366
Anesthesia equipment, 264
Aseptic technique, 360
Association for the Advancement of Medical Instrumentation
    flash sterilization recommendations of, 292, 296
    packaging systems recommendations of, 266
    reprocessing report of, 374
    standards of, 292, 296
    steam sterilization monitoring recommendations of, 328
Association of Perioperative Registered Nurses (AORN)
    chemical indicator recommendations of, 331
    flash sterilization recommendations of, 292, 294–295
    infection control policy statement of, 356–367
    packaging system recommendations of, 266
    policy statement of, 328
    reprocessing statement of, 380–381
    standards of, 351
    sterilization recommendations of, 266
Association of Professionals in Infection Control, 351

B

Bioburden, removal of, for infection prevention, 359
Biofilm, removal of, for infection prevention, 359
Biological indicators
    for flash sterilization, 310–311, 315–316
    for steam sterilization, 336
Bowie-Dick test
    for flash sterilization, 308–310
    for steam sterilization, 275–276, 331
Brain tissue, contamination with, special considerations for, 278–279

C

Cataract surgery, toxic anterior segment syndrome in, 298, 300–302, 399–401
Centers for Disease Control and Prevention, inspections by, 348–351

Perioperative Nursing Clinics 5 (2010) 401–409
doi:10.1016/S1556-7931(10)00057-4
1556-7931/10/$ – see front matter © 2010 Elsevier Inc. All rights reserved.

periopnursing.theclinics.com